Where's
my spatula?

Where's my spatula?

**Fast, Healthy Meals
When Your Kitchen or
Your Life Is a Mess**

CHRISTY ROST

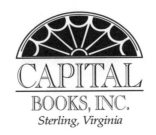

CAPITAL
BOOKS, INC.
Sterling, Virginia

Capital Books, Inc.
P.O. Box 605
Herndon, Virginia 20172-0605

ISBN 13: 978-1-933102-67-2

Library of Congress Cataloging-in-Publication Data
Library of Congress Cataloging-in-Publication Data

Rost, Christy.
Where's my spatula? : fast, healthy meals when your kitchen or your life is a mess / Christy Rost. — 1st ed.
p. cm.
ISBN 978-1-933102-67-2 (alk. paper)
1. Cookery. I. Title.

TX714.R6754 2008
641.5—dc22

2008000098

Printed in the United States of America on acid-free paper that meets the American National Standards Institute Z39-48 Standard.

First Edition

10 9 8 7 6 5 4 3 2 1

To Randy, my sweet husband
and gifted house remodeler.
Thank you for buying me the home in
the mountains we've always dreamed of.
May it always be filled with love, family,
friends, celebration, and great food!

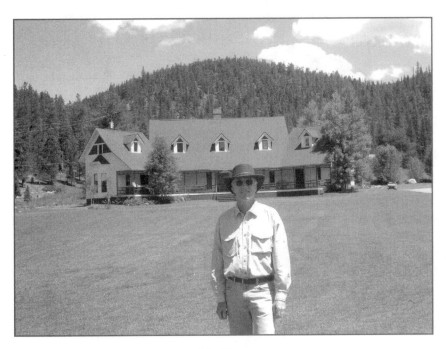

My Hero

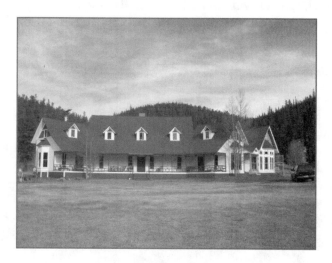

Swan's Nest
Swan's Nest under construction.

contents

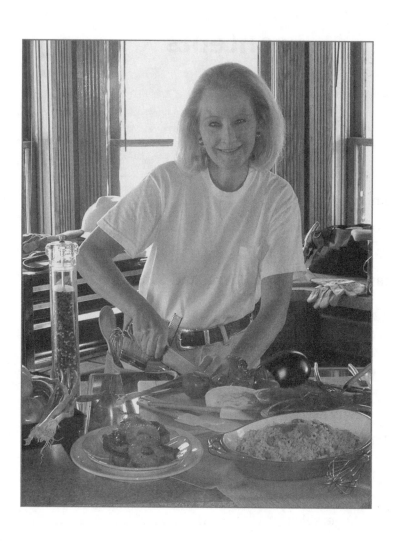

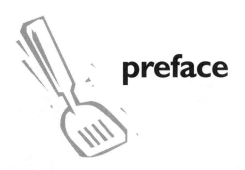

preface

Writing and developing recipes for *Where's My Spatula?* has presented special challenges. Instead of my spacious, well-equipped home kitchen in Dallas, Texas, I have worked in a postage stamp-size kitchen in Dillon, Colorado. I've learned to cook and bake at high altitude, and my office has been the kitchen table or living room sofa and coffee table. Certainly not the ideal circumstances for a cookbook author!

I've also written this book in the midst of a major historic house restoration. Each day has been filled to the brim with attending meetings, making decisions, sweeping up construction dust, hauling dirt to create new gardens, selecting new windows, doors, paint colors, and fireplace mantels, pouring over designs for the new master bath and kitchen addition, and finding amazing historical discoveries hidden behind the walls. It's been an exciting, joyous, and demanding time.

These challenges have provided me opportunities to develop recipes with my readers in mind. I've learned to simplify my cooking without sacrificing quality or taste. I experienced what many experience every day—not enough time or energy to cook at the end of the day—and yet, I still managed to join my husband, Randy, at the table each evening over a tasty, nutritious meal shared in flickering candlelight, created in a matter of minutes, not hours.

As you, the reader, cook from these pages, it is my hope you will find recipes that inspire and nourish you, ease that end-of-the-day stress, and provide easy mealtime solutions. May you always know where your spatula is.

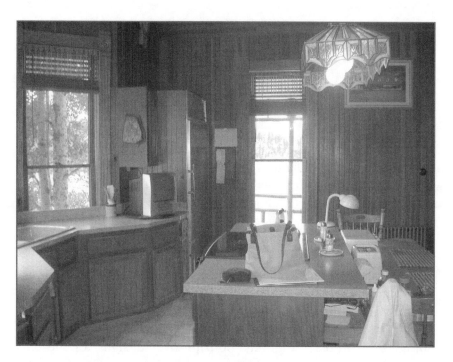

The Old Kitchen
This room was originally Ben Revett's office, with an adjacent gold vault where Ben stored his gold. Beautiful 110-year-old fir paneling covers the walls and ceiling, making the kitchen dark and uninviting. My challenge is to transform this dated room into a warm, welcoming kitchen.

acknowledgments

I would like to express very special thanks to my mother-in-law, Pat Rost Shilstone, who generously and lovingly gave us the use of her condominium in Dillon, Colorado, for the entire summer, so Randy and I could restore our historic home and I could write this cookbook. She's always been a great supporter of my work—I call her my PR agent—and I'm so lucky to have her as my "mom."

Thanks also go to Liz and Al Wickert, our new Breckenridge, Colorado, neighbors and sweet friends who live next door to Swan's Nest. Both are highly gifted cooks and generous hosts, and Randy and I were their guests many times while I wrote this book. Their enthusiasm and passion for great food have inspired me to stretch my culinary wings, and their warmth and friendship have made me feel very much at home in our new mountain neighborhood.

And, finally, a heartfelt thank you to my publisher, Kathleen Hughes, at Capital Books. She has believed in my approach to "cooking with love" from the first time we spoke and has eagerly awaited this book. Kathleen, you definitely rate five spatulas!

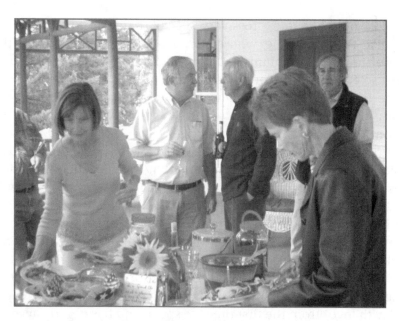

Keep It Simple

Entertaining is easy when you keep it simple. For our Labor Day picnic on the porch, Randy and I cooked out on the grill and guests each brought a dish. Coolers were filled with ice cold drinks,

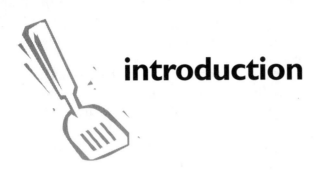

introduction

Developing recipes and writing a cookbook while restoring an historic home is not the way I envisioned my next cookbook project, but since "overload" seems to be the standard by which many of us live these days, perhaps it's not as absurd as it sounds. *Where's My Spatula?* was inspired by my present circumstances: the need to prepare fast, healthy meals when each day is filled to the brim with office hours, contractor meetings, problem solving; fixture, color, and texture selection; and decision making, such as choosing whether to delay the start of our new kitchen addition until spring or to begin the work in late summer and risk damage by an early winter snowstorm before the structure is enclosed.

My husband, Randy, and I discovered our house (Randy refers to it as "the project") just over a year ago while looking for property for a vacation home in the Breckenridge area of Colorado. Built in 1898 by Ben Stanley Revett, "the gold dredge king," the structure sits on fourteen gorgeous acres at the base of the Ten Mile Range in the Rocky Mountains. We are only the third family to own the house, a fact I find rather remarkable, but during its 109-year history, it has served as a hunting lodge and as a camp for kids—twice! These rather odd uses, plus a partial renovation in the 1970s, have left their mark on the once-grand home. Randy and I are restoring it to the gracious home it deserves to be, and we are also restoring its original name, Swan's Nest.

Despite lacking running water and having nothing but extension cords for power, Randy and I have managed to cook lunch for our construction crew on numerous occasions—there's no worker like a well-fed worker!—thanks to an inexpensive charcoal grill and coolers, to keep ingredients well-chilled. We've grilled in the rain and gusty winds and on gorgeous sunny days, surrounded by majestic mountain peaks that have me pinching myself now and then to be sure it's all real.

Randy and I have also entertained our new friends and neighbors at Swan's Nest. Our first three dinner parties were held on the expansive front porch because most of the rooms have been littered with power and hand tools, hundred-year-old wood we carefully removed and labeled for storage until we are ready to replace it, and the ever-present lack of electricity. In fact, in preparation for one of our late-afternoon parties, I wrapped the porch railings with white holiday lights attached to two extension cords, just in case the party lasted into the evening. In the end, Randy and I packed up dishes, glassware, and leftovers by the light of the porch railing and packed it all into the car for the trip back to our tiny condo, where we washed all the dishes. And, no, we did not use paper plates. We may not have electricity and running water yet, but we always dine with our friends in style.

On many evenings Randy and I have arrived back at our little condo after a day at the house, exhausted and hungry, with no prior thoughts of dinner. Some may not be able to imagine how a quick search of the refrigerator and pantry can yield a delicious meal in a matter of minutes, but I know the key to fast, nourishing meals is lots of fresh ingredients in the fridge and a few staples in the cupboard. I'm also a big believer in leftovers. When I sauté chicken breast halves for a quick dinner, I always sauté four, instead of the two I need for that evening. Those extra cooked chicken breasts give me a head start on dinner the following night, whether sliced for a chilled main dish salad or quickly sautéed in olive oil with a dash of cumin and fresh cilantro and rolled into flour tortillas with crisp Romaine lettuce and zesty salsa.

One element not found in my previous cookbook, *The Family Table*, was a pantry list. A significant number of readers requested I add a list in my next book, so you'll be happy to know I've included a section in this cookbook called "A Well-Stocked Kitchen." A pantry stocked with your favorite items can eliminate countless last-minute trips to the supermarket, thus saving precious time and gas money, and can even be the source of inspiration for spur-of-the-moment recipes. I also think just knowing there's a pantry full of mouthwatering, good-for-you ingredients is reason enough to bypass the fast-food establishments on the way home from work or errands. After all, what fried chicken place can compete with oven-baked molasses barbecued chicken or mostaccioli pasta and spinach with freshly grated Pecorino Romano cheese, accompanied by a loaf of rustic bread with an olive oil, balsamic vinegar, and Parmesan dipping sauce?

I regard my pantry as a mini corner grocery store that specializes in all my favorite ingredients—a variety of vinegars so I can whip up a dressing or dipping sauce without giving it a second's thought, good quality olive oil, and canned goods that help me "zip up" an everyday salad or create a sumptuous pasta dinner in thirty minutes when I forgot to take something out of the freezer to defrost that morning.

In addition to the pantry, I've made a list of items I typically stock in my refrigerator, freezer, and spice cabinet. Fabulous, good-for-you meals that bring families to the table day after day depend on more than dried pasta and canned goods. Fresh ingredients are important elements of good nutrition and flavorful meals that keep everyone coming back to the table, without stopping in the fast-food lane on the way home. In addition to the usual milk, eggs, and butter, my refrigerator always contains fresh, seasonal fruits and vegetables, fresh herbs to add a burst of flavor to meals, flour tortillas—one can do so many things with a tortilla for breakfast, lunch, or dinner—and a selection of both hard and soft cheeses.

In the freezer, I keep a ready supply of meats, fish, and seafood. Boneless chicken breasts are one of my staples. After removing the skin, I can sauté, bake, stir-fry, or grill the breasts and have a tasty, healthy meal on the table within thirty to forty minutes. When dinnertime arrives and I've forgotten to take meat out of the freezer, I know frozen shrimp can be defrosted in cold water in a matter of minutes. By the time I hang up my coat and set the table, the shrimp are just about ready to toss into a pan with olive oil, garlic, and a few herbs. Served with a vegetable and a salad or side dish, shrimp can make up a complete meal even on the most hectic days.

Whether you're remodeling, moving, working nonstop, juggling a career, child care, and home all at the same time, or caring for someone who is ill, you have no doubt had moments when the thought of cooking a meal at the end of a busy day left you panicky. Where in the world will you find the energy to spend an hour in the kitchen preparing dinner?

What should you do? Drive through the take-out line? Call out for pizza again, or maybe Chinese? What about your vow to eat healthier meals? What about your *budget*? Ordering takeout or driving through the fast-food lane often isn't the healthy choice when it comes to quick meals and can be expensive. We're all aware that home cooking with fresh ingredients is the best method for a healthy lifestyle, but how can you fit cooking into the day when you're already stressed out?

Take a deep breath and open my newest cookbook, *Where's My Spatula? Fast, Healthy Meals When Your Kitchen or Your Life Is a Mess.* Herein, you will find answers to your dinner dilemma—nutritious, delicious recipes that can be prepared quickly and with minimum fuss. Best of all, you and your family will love these meals. In the pages of this book are recipes to help you eat well without resorting to fast food. You'll even find recipes for quick desserts because, face it, most of us crave something sweet now and then. The key to a healthy diet is to enjoy a small dessert serving and share the rest! So, cancel that carry-out order, head straight for home, and grab your spatula. Dinner is almost on the table.

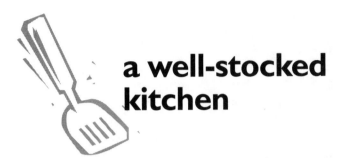

a well-stocked kitchen

pantry

Baking chocolate, semi-sweet
Baking chocolate, unsweetened
Baking powder
Baking soda
Balsamic vinegar
Brown sugar
Canned black beans
Canned diced tomatoes
Canned garbanzo beans
Canned pineapple rings
Canned quartered artichoke hearts
Canned tomato sauce
Capers
Cornstarch
Dried cranberries
Dry red wine
Dry white wine
Flour
Garlic
Kosher salt or sea salt
Low-fat beef broth
Low-fat chicken broth
No-cook lasagna noodles

where's my spatula?

Olive oil
Olives, black and green
Onions, red and sweet
Parchment paper
Pasta
   Linguini
   Penne
   Spaghetti
   Whole-wheat pasta
   Wide noodles
Peppercorns, black and multi-color mélange
Picante sauce or salsa
Quick-cooking rolled oats
Raisins
Red potatoes
Red wine vinegar
Rice
   Brown rice
   Jasmine rice
   Long-grain rice
Rice vinegar
Roasted red sweet peppers (in jar)
Shallots
Sugar, confectioners' and granulated
Sweet potatoes
Vanilla extract
Vine-ripened tomatoes
Worcestershire sauce

refrigerator

Apple cider or juice
Apples
Bell peppers, assorted colors
Bok choy
Butter, unsalted
Carrots

Celery
Cheese
  Aged Parmesan cheese
  Feta cheese, crumbled
  Goat cheese
  Monterey Jack cheese
  Mozzarella
  Pecorino Romano cheese
Dijon mustard
Eggs
Flour tortillas
Grapes
Heavy cream
Herbs
  Fresh basil
  Fresh cilantro
  Fresh oregano
  Fresh parsley
  Fresh rosemary
Lemons
Lettuce, leaf or Romaine
Low-fat milk
Mayonnaise
Nonfat plain yogurt
Nonfat sour cream
Oranges
Seasonal fruit
Seasonal vegetables

freezer

Boneless chicken breasts
Fish
Ground chuck
Lamb chops
Lamb stew meat
Pork chops
Puff pastry sheets
Sea scallops
Shrimp, raw, peeled, and deveined
Sirloin steak

dried herbs and spices

Basil
Bay leaves
Chili powder
Cinnamon
Cumin
Garlic powder
Onion powder
Oregano
Paprika
Red pepper flakes
Rosemary
Sage
Tarragon
Thyme
Whole nutmeg

meats, seafood, pasta, pizza, and sandwiches

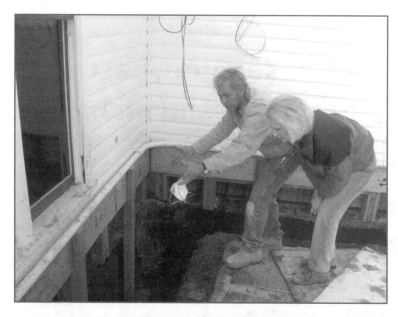

I Promise The House Won't Fall

When the back hallway drops 6 inches from one end to the other, it's a pretty good indication there's a foundation problem. Here, our master carpenter Larry explains how 100-year-old timbers rotted from years of moisture, and the solution he devised to support Swan's Nest until the foundation company could make repairs. I'm sure our neighbors thought we were moving the house!

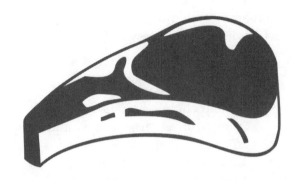

meats

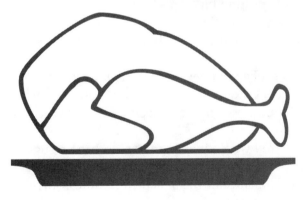

oven-baked molasses barbecued chicken breasts

One of the easiest recipes I know is oven-baked chicken breasts. Brush on my sweet but tangy sauce that's ready in less than 15 minutes, and you'll have an easy meal that's dripping with flavor. Try the molasses sauce on your favorite chicken pieces, from drumsticks to wings, and transform an ordinary weekday dinner into a fun family gathering. There's no need to stand in the carry-out line when dinner's this easy.

Ingredients:
1 tablespoon canola oil
1/2 cup chopped onion
2 large cloves garlic, peeled and minced
2/3 cup ketchup
1 1/2 tablespoons red wine vinegar
1 tablespoon molasses
1 tablespoon brown sugar
1/4 teaspoon Worcestershire sauce
1/4 teaspoon freshly ground black pepper
3–4 drops Tabasco sauce, optional
4 to 6 skinless chicken breasts, bone-in or boneless

Preheat a medium saucepan over medium-low heat, add the canola oil, and swirl to coat the bottom of the pan. Add the onion and garlic, and sauté 3 minutes, stirring occasionally, until the onions are softened.

Stir in the ketchup, red wine vinegar, molasses, brown sugar, Worcestershire sauce, pepper, and Tabasco sauce, if desired. Reduce the heat to low and simmer the sauce 10 minutes, stirring occasionally.

Preheat the oven to 350°F. Arrange the chicken pieces in a large baking pan, brush them generously with some of the sauce, and cover the pan tightly with foil. Bake 40 to 50 minutes, until the chicken is tender, brushing pieces occasionally with the remaining sauce.

Yield: 4 to 6 servings

chicken breasts, fennel, and sweet potatoes in parchment paper

Cooking in parchment paper shouldn't be reserved for seafood because it works really well for chicken, too. In this recipe, I've paired boneless chicken breasts with fennel bulb and sweet potatoes, and spiced the combo up with garlic, onion, sage, and bay leaf. After the packet steams in the oven, its contents are moist, tender, and flavorful, and there's virtually no cleanup. This is a great meal for a busy night.

Ingredients:
2 (18-inch) lengths parchment paper
2 boneless, skinless chicken breasts
1 cup peeled and cubed fresh sweet potato
1/2 teaspoon garlic powder
1/2 teaspoon onion powder
1/2 teaspoon dried sage
1/2 cup chopped red onion
1 cup chopped fresh fennel
4 sprigs fresh parsley, chopped
2 bay leaves

Preheat the oven to 350°F. Spread 2 sheets of parchment paper out on a roasting pan or cookie sheet. Center each chicken breast on a sheet of parchment and surround it with sweet potato cubes. Sprinkle the meat with the garlic powder, onion powder, sage, onion, fennel, and parsley, and place a bay leaf on top of each chicken breast.

Gather up the edges of the parchment paper, fold them down twice, and twist the ends securely to seal in the meat. Bake the packets for 30 minutes, or until the meat is tender and the sweet potatoes and fennel are knife tender.

Transfer the parchment packets to two dinner plates, unfold, and serve.

Yield: 2 servings

chicken piccata

Simple but elegant, this Italian classic can transform a hectic evening into an enjoyable interlude. Add candlelight and you have the ingredients for a quiet meal with the family or a romantic dinner for two. The chicken's crisp exterior and the lemon wine sauce are sublime. When you have only a few minutes to get a meal on the table, trust me, this recipe is for you.

Ingredients:
4 boneless, skinless chicken breast halves
1/2 cup flour
1/2 teaspoon salt
1/4 teaspoon freshly ground black pepper
1 tablespoon olive oil
1 tablespoon unsalted butter
3/4 cup chicken stock or broth
1/2 cup dry white wine
1 lemon, halved and thinly sliced
1/3 cup sliced black olives
1 tablespoon capers, rinsed and drained

Rinse the chicken breasts and dry them on paper towels. Place each chicken breast between sheets of plastic wrap on a cutting board and pound them with a meat mallet or cast-iron skillet to 1/2 inch thickness; set aside.

Preheat a large skillet over medium heat. While the skillet is heating, stir together the flour, salt, and pepper in a large shallow bowl or plate. Dredge each chicken breast in the flour mixture, add the olive oil and butter to the skillet, and place the chicken in the skillet. Cook the meat until it is golden brown on one side, about 3 minutes. Turn it over and cook 2 to 3 minutes more, or until it is golden brown.

When the meat is done, transfer it to a serving platter and keep it warm. Deglaze the pan with chicken stock and wine, stirring well to scrape up brown bits. Add lemon slices and cook until the liquid is reduced by half. Return the meat to the skillet and stir in the black olives and capers. Cook 2 minutes and serve.

Yield: 4 servings

turkey sausage and rice skillet

When you're trying to get a nutritious dinner on the table with minimum fuss, this one-skillet meal is the answer. Turkey sausage, rice, chopped bell pepper, onion, diced tomatoes, and canned green chiles are simmered with dried herbs and spices for a mouth-tingling, satisfying skillet casserole that's quick and easy.

Ingredients:
1 cup chicken stock or broth
1 cup water
1 cup converted or long-grain rice
1 yellow or green bell pepper, seeded and chopped
3/4 cup chopped onion
3 large cloves garlic, peeled and chopped
1 (14.5-ounce) can petite diced tomatoes
1 (4.5-ounce) can diced green chiles, drained
1 (14-ounce) package turkey smoked sausage
1 teaspoon Italian seasoning
1/2 teaspoon cumin
1/2 teaspoon anise seed, ground with a mortar and pestle
1/2 teaspoon coarse salt
Generous grinding of black pepper
3 tablespoons fresh sage, chopped

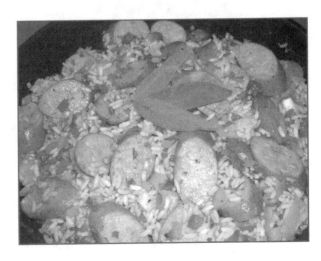

Pour the chicken broth and water into a large cast-iron skillet, add the rice, and bring to a boil over high heat. Reduce the heat to medium-low, cover, and cook the rice about 15 minutes, or until most of the liquid is absorbed.

Add the bell pepper, onion, and garlic, and cook the mixture 2 to 3 minutes, stirring frequently, until the pepper and aromatics begin to soften. Stir in the tomatoes, green chiles, sausage, Italian seasoning, cumin, anise, salt, and pepper. Cover the skillet and cook the mixture over medium-low heat 10 to 15 minutes, or until the casserole is hot. Add the sage, stir, and cook 2 minutes more.

Serve the casserole directly from the skillet, or spoon it into a serving bowl and serve immediately.

Yield: 6 servings

grilled sirloin with sage derby cheese

With its attractive mantle of green and white cheese, melted and swirled during the final minutes of grilling, this dish is the perfect entrée for St. Patrick's Day, but it's so delicious, you'll want to serve it year round. The creamy texture and buttery, fresh sage flavor of sage Derby cheese from Ireland provides this dish with both color and savoriness. If you can't find sage Derby cheese in your local market, experiment with other cheeses and create your own taste and visual experience.

1 1/4 pound sirloin steak, about 1/2 inch thickness
Coarse salt and freshly ground black pepper, to taste
2 ounces sage Derby cheese, sliced

Preheat the grill. While the grill is heating, season the steak with salt and pepper.

Place the steak on the grill once it has preheated and cook 3 to 4 minutes. Turn the meat over and cook 3 to 4 minutes more, or until the steak is brown on the outside and almost done. Flip the meat again and cook 1 to 2 minutes more on each side for medium-rare doneness, rotating the meat to create nice grill marks.

During the final 1 to 2 minutes of cooking, arrange cheese slices on top of the meat, and close the grill cover. The cheese will melt and produce a swirled mantle over the meat.

Transfer the meat to a serving platter, let it rest several minutes to draw in its juices, and serve.

Yield: 4 servings

beef and vegetable skewers with hoisin barbecue sauce

I created this dish one afternoon when we had invited friends over for dinner. They knew from the start they were going to be guinea pigs for the evening, tasting new recipes for inclusion in this book. The skewers were an instant sensation. Not only did they look impressive piled on the platter, hot from the grill, but their flavor was fabulous. You'll be happy to know the vote was unanimous: this recipe was a keeper! On busy days, purchase ready-made ka-bobs at your local supermarket and brush them with my quick and easy hoisin barbecue sauce.

Ingredients:
1 tablespoon canola oil
1/4 cup sweet onion, minced
2 large cloves garlic, peeled and minced
1 cup hoisin sauce
3 tablespoons rice vinegar
2 tablespoons ketchup
1 tablespoon soy sauce
1 tablespoon sake rice wine
1 tablespoon brown sugar, packed
5 to 6 drops Tabasco sauce
4 to 5 drops Worcestershire sauce
1/4 teaspoon crushed red pepper flakes
2 pounds beef loin top sirloin, cut into 2-inch cubes
1 1/2 large sweet onions, cut into wedges
1 green bell pepper, cut into wedges
1 red bell pepper, cut into wedges
2 yellow squash, sliced into 1-inch pieces
2 zucchini, sliced into 1-inch pieces
2 dozen cherry tomatoes
12 long metal skewers

Preheat a medium saucepan over medium heat, add the canola oil, and swirl to coat the bottom of the pan. Add the onion and garlic, stir, and sauté 2 minutes until the onions begin to soften. Stir in the hoisin sauce, rice vinegar, ketchup, soy sauce, sake, brown sugar, Tabasco, Worcestershire, and red pepper flakes. Reduce the heat to low and simmer the sauce 15 to 20 minutes, stirring occasionally. (Sauce may be made one day ahead, chilled, and reheated just before grilling.)

Thread beef cubes, onion, bell peppers, yellow squash, zucchini, and cherry tomatoes alternately onto the skewers.

Preheat the grill to medium heat. When the grill is hot, place half of the skewers on the grill and cook them 12 to 15 minutes, turning them occasionally. During the final 5 minutes of cooking time, brush the meat and vegetables generously with some of the hoisin sauce.

Transfer the cooked skewers to a platter and cover them to keep them warm. Grill the remaining skewers as above. Serve them on a bed of couscous or flavored rice.

Yield: 12 beef skewers, or 8 to 12 servings

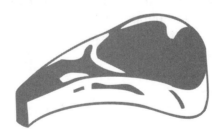

savory skillet beef and broccoli

When dinner has to be fast, this savory dish really hits the spot. Tender slices of beef are quickly sautéed with crisp-tender broccoli florets and a rich broth for a meal that's quick, flavorful, and nutritious. Serve the beef and broccoli with couscous, rice, or noodles for a complete meal.

Ingredients:
2 tablespoons olive oil
1 pound beef sirloin, sliced into thin strips
3 cups broccoli florets
2 large cloves garlic, peeled and minced
1/4 cup dry red wine
1/2 cup beef stock or broth
1 tablespoon tomato paste
3 drops Worcestershire sauce
Coarse salt and freshly ground black pepper, to taste

Preheat a large skillet over medium heat, add the olive oil, and swirl to coat the bottom of the pan. Add the beef, cook until it browns on the bottom, and turn it over to cook on the other side. Transfer the beef to a medium bowl and keep it warm.

Add the broccoli florets and minced garlic to the skillet and sauté 1 minute. Add the wine, beef stock, tomato paste, and Worcestershire and stir to blend. Return the beef to the skillet, season with salt and pepper, and cook 2 minutes more. Serve with couscous, rice, or noodles, if desired.

Yield: 4 servings

teriyaki cashew beef stir-fry

After a full day of house restoration projects, I stirred up this flavorful dish in an ordinary skillet and had dinner on the table in 30 minutes. For variety, add your favorite vegetables or what's freshest in the market. For this stir-fry you can also use leftover meat from a steak, roasted chicken, or pork roast dinner. Just stir-fry the vegetables, add sauce and thinly sliced leftover meat, and cook until the meat is heated through. It's faster than take-out, and your family will love it.

Ingredients:
1 pound boneless beef top sirloin
2 tablespoons canola oil, divided
1/2 pound broccoli crowns, trimmed and cut
   into bite-size pieces
1/4 pound pea pods, stems removed
1/2 cup cashews
1 tablespoon cornstarch
2 tablespoons soy sauce
2 tablespoons sake or sherry
2 tablespoons beef broth
1 tablespoon honey
2 teaspoons brown sugar, packed
1 teaspoon freshly grated gingerroot or
   1/2 teaspoon dried ginger
Steamed rice

Slice the beef into 1/4-inch-thick bite-size strips and set aside. Preheat a wok or large skillet over medium-high heat, add 1 tablespoon of the oil, and swirl to coat the bottom of the pan. Add half of the beef and stir-fry until it is just cooked through, about 1 minute. Transfer the meat to a bowl, quickly stir-fry the remaining beef, and transfer it to the bowl.

Add the remaining oil to the pan and stir-fry the broccoli, pea pods, and cashews until the vegetables are crisp-tender. In a small bowl, stir together the cornstarch, soy sauce, sake, beef broth, honey, brown sugar, and gingerroot. Pour the sauce into the pan and stir. Add cooked beef, and cook 1 minute, stirring frequently. Serve over steamed rice.

Yield: 4 servings

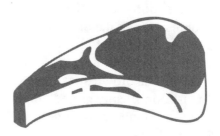

fifteen-minute pork chops with cabernet reduction

This deluxe pork chop recipe makes it possible to have gourmet flavor and still get dinner on the table in 15 minutes. I developed this recipe, after a long, hectic day of working on our historic house with my husband. Randy and I were hungry and tired, and stopping at the supermarket was *not* an option. A quick search of our tiny condo kitchen revealed four pork rib chops, an open bottle of Cabernet, and fresh garlic—the makings of a feast. Fifteen minutes later, we sat down to a candlelit dinner.

Ingredients:
4 pork loin rib chops, about 3/4 inch thickness
Coarse salt and freshly ground pepper, to taste
1 tablespoon olive oil
3 cloves garlic, diced
1/3 cup Cabernet or other dry red wine
1/2 cup beef broth or stock
1 teaspoon dried rosemary, crushed between hands
1/8 teaspoon rubbed sage
1 tablespoon unsalted butter, softened

Preheat a large skillet over medium heat. Season the chops with salt and pepper. Add oil to the skillet, swirl to coat the bottom of the pan, and add the chops. Cook 5 minutes until the meat is brown, turn the chops over, and cook 5 to 7 minutes more, depending on their thickness.

Transfer the meat to a serving platter and cover it with foil to keep warm. Drain all fat from the skillet, add garlic, and sauté 1 minute, stirring constantly. Deglaze the pan with wine and beef broth, stirring to loosen brown bits from the skillet. Add dried rosemary and sage. Bring the wine sauce to a boil and cook several minutes until it is reduced by half. Remove the skillet from the heat, and if desired, stir in cold butter to thicken and flavor the sauce. Season the sauce with salt and pepper, and spoon it over the pork chops.

Yield: 4 servings

grilled pork chops with wasabi ginger marinade

These grilled boneless pork chops are absolutely delicious and so quick and easy. The marinade features soy sauce and brown sugar with a touch of Japanese wasabi horseradish and ground ginger, which when grilled, provides a mouth-pleasing array of flavors.

Ingredients:
1/2 cup soy sauce
1 tablespoon brown sugar, packed
1/2 teaspoon wasabi horseradish paste
1/4 teaspoon ground ginger
1 1/2 pounds pork loin boneless chops
Freshly ground black pepper, to taste

Preheat the grill. In a large shallow bowl, stir together the soy sauce, brown sugar, wasabi paste, and ginger until they are well blended.

Season the pork chops with pepper and place them in the marinade 15 to 30 minutes, turning them over several times. When the grill is hot, transfer the meat to a platter and pour the marinade into a small saucepan. Bring the marinade to a boil over high heat, reduce the heat to low, and simmer 5 minutes.

Place the meat on the grill and cook 3 to 4 minutes, basting occasionally with the hot marinade. Turn the chops over and cook 3 to 4 minutes more, basting occasionally. Turn the meat again and cook 2 to 3 minutes more, or until it is done, rotating the pieces on the grill to create nice grill marks. Remove the meat from the grill and serve immediately.

Yield: 4 servings.

pork chops with spiced apples

This succulent dish features two of my autumn favorites—pork chops and apples. Tender, juicy bone-in pork chops are sautéed in a cast-iron skillet and topped with sliced apples that have been cooked in an apple cider, cinnamon, and garlic reduction sauce. The balance of savory and sweet is satisfying and delicious, and best of all, this recipe is ready in 30 minutes.

Ingredients:
Coarse salt and freshly ground black pepper; to taste
2 to 4 bone-in pork loin chops, about 1/2 inch thickness
2 large cloves garlic, peeled and minced
1/2 cup apple cider
1/4 cup chicken stock or broth
2 apples, peeled, cored, and sliced
1/8 teaspoon cinnamon
1/8 teaspoon freshly grated nutmeg

Sprinkle a large cast-iron skillet over medium heat with 1/8 teaspoon salt. Season the pork chops on both sides with salt and pepper and place them in the pan. Cook them 3 to 4 minutes, or until they are brown on the bottom. Turn them over and cook them 3 to 4 minutes more to brown the other side. Turn and cook the chops 2 additional minutes on each side, transfer them to a plate, and cover them to keep them warm.

Add garlic to the pan and sauté 1 minute until it is soft. Deglaze the pan with apple cider and chicken stock, stirring to loosen brown bits from the bottom of the pan. Stir in the apples, cinnamon, and nutmeg, and cook 5 minutes, until the apples start to soften and the liquid is reduced by half.

Return the pork chops to the pan, season them lightly with salt and pepper, cover, and reduce the heat to low. Cook the chops 10 to 15 minutes or until the meat is cooked through and the apples are tender. To serve, arrange pork chops on a serving platter and spoon the apples and remaining sauce over the meat.

Yield: 2 to 4 servings.

breaded pork cutlets with creamy horseradish sauce

Thinly sliced boneless pork chops are dipped in egg and a corn-meal flour mixture in this quick and tasty busy-day recipe. After sautéing, the cutlets are moist and tender inside, with a golden, crisp layer of breading on the outside. Served with a creamy horseradish sauce you can stir up in two minutes, it's a deliciously simple week-day meal.

Ingredients:
1/4 cup low-fat sour cream
1 tablespoon mayonnaise
2 to 3 teaspoons prepared horseradish
1/2 teaspoon plus a dash of coarse salt, divided
1/2 cup flour
1/4 cup cornmeal
1/4 teaspoon garlic powder
1/4 teaspoon onion powder
Freshly ground black pepper, to taste
1 egg
1 1/4 pounds thin-sliced pork loin sirloin boneless chops
2 to 3 tablespoons olive oil

In a small bowl, stir together sour cream, mayonnaise, horse-radish, and a dash of salt until they are well blended. Spoon into a serving bowl and set aside. (Leftover sauce may be covered and chilled up to 3 days.)

In a large plastic zipper bag, place flour, cornmeal, the remaining 1/2 teaspoon salt, garlic powder, onion powder, and pepper. Seal the bag and shake well to mix.

Preheat a large skillet over medium heat. In a small bowl, whip the egg with a fork until it is light. Dip the pork cutlets into the egg and drop them into the bag of flour mixture, one or two at a time, seal the bag, and shake until the cutlets are well coated. If desired, dip the coated cutlets into the egg and coat them in the flour mixture a second time.

Add 2 tablespoons of the olive oil to the skillet, swirl to coat the bottom of the pan, and place the cutlets in the pan. Sauté them 4 to 5 minutes until the breading is golden brown, turn them over, and sauté 4 to 5 minutes more, or until the meat is done. If the cutlets start to stick to the bottom of the skillet, add the remaining olive oil. Transfer the cutlets to a platter and serve with horseradish sauce.

Yield: 4 servings

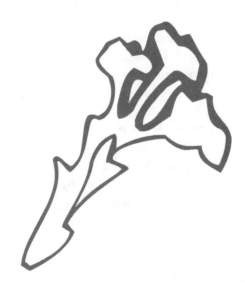

barbecued hawaiian pork ribs with sweet, hot, and sour sauce

Have plenty of napkins handy while enjoying these sensational ribs. The sauce is everything you could desire—sweet, spicy, and tangy all at the same time. Braising the meat in the oven breaks down its collagen, which makes it tender even before you finish it on the grill. While this recipe may not be your best choice for quick mealtime preparation, I *had* to include it for weekend barbecues. Once you try these ribs, you'll be glad I did.

Ingredients:
5 pounds rack of pork
1 cup ketchup
1/4 cup pineapple juice
2 tablespoons brown sugar, packed
2 tablespoons rice vinegar
1 tablespoon chili garlic sauce
3 drops Worcestershire sauce
Freshly ground peppercorn mélange
Canned or fresh pineapple rings, for garnish

Preheat the oven to 350°F. Place the pork ribs in a large roasting pan, slicing the rack in half if it is too long to fit in the pan. Pour water into the pan to a depth of 1/4 inch, cover it tightly with foil, and braise the ribs in a preheated oven 45 minutes.

While the ribs cook, or one day ahead, prepare the barbecue sauce. In a medium saucepan, stir together the ketchup, pineapple juice, brown sugar, rice vinegar, chili garlic sauce, Worcestershire sauce, and peppercorn mélange. Cook over medium heat, stirring occasionally, until the sauce comes to a low boil. Reduce the heat to low and cook 30 minutes more, stirring occasionally.

Preheat the grill. When it is hot, reduce the heat to low, remove the ribs from the roasting pan and place them on the grill, meat side down. Baste them with some of the barbecue sauce and cook 15 minutes. Turn them over and baste with more of the sauce. Cook the ribs 30 to 40 minutes more, basting occasionally with the sauce, until they are tender and the meat releases from the ends of the bones.

Yield: 4 to 6 servings

slow-cooked home-style pork roast stew

When I was married, more than a few years ago, Crock-Pots were a popular wedding gift. My husband, Randy, and I used ours now and again for a couple of years until it found its way to the back of a cupboard. Recently, as our lives have become busier, Crock-Pots have reemerged with a new name and a wealth of flavorful recipe suggestions. Today's slow cookers are larger and more versatile, and they can be a valuable solution to the problem of getting a nutritious, delicious meal on the table with a minimum of time and effort. My recipe for pork roast stew is large on flavor and specially designed for today's slow cookers.

Ingredients:
1 (6-pound) pork butt roast
3 tablespoons olive oil, divided
1 cup dry red wine, divided
3 stalks celery, sliced
1 bunch fresh celery leaves
1 large onion, peeled and coarsely chopped
1 head garlic, peeled and coarsely chopped
2 pounds small red potatoes, rinsed
1 (14.5-ounce) can diced tomatoes
3/4 cup chicken or beef stock or broth
2 sprigs fresh rosemary
1 bay leaf
1 teaspoon herbes de Provence
Freshly ground black pepper, to taste

Cut the pork butt into 3-inch pieces, trimming the fat as needed. Preheat a large skillet over medium heat, add 1 tablespoon of the olive oil, and swirl to coat the bottom of the pan. Place one-third of the meat in the skillet, cook it several minutes on each side, until it is brown, and transfer it to the slow cooker.

Deglaze the pan with 1/3 cup of the red wine, scraping up brown bits from the bottom of the skillet with a rubber spatula or wooden spoon, and pour the wine mixture into the slow cooker. Repeat the process with the next 2 batches of meat and the remaining red wine.

When all the meat has been browned and transferred to the slow cooker, add the celery, celery leaves, onion, garlic, and potatoes to the meat mixture. Pour in the tomatoes and chicken stock, and season with the rosemary, bay leaf, herbes de Provence, and pepper.

Cover, set the slow cooker on low heat, and set the timer for 4 to 5 hours. After 4 hours, check the meat and potatoes for tenderness by piercing them with a sharp knife. The meat should almost fall apart, and the knife should penetrate the potatoes easily. Turn the cooker to the warm setting until ready to serve.

Yield: 6 to 8 servings

fruit-glazed ham steaks

Now you can have the flavor of a large holiday ham with the convenience of ham loaf for everyday enjoyment. Thick slices of ham are garnished with a spicy brown sugar and molasses fruit sauce, enriched with dried apricots and cranberries, chunks of pineapple, raisins, and cherries. This dish is so attractive, you'll want to serve it when entertaining.

Ingredients:
1 (4-pound) ham loaf, sliced into 1/4-inch-thick slices
1 1/2 cups peach nectar
1/4 cup brown sugar, packed
1/2 teaspoon molasses
1/4 teaspoon ground cloves
1/8 teaspoon cinnamon
1 1/4 cups dried apricots
1 (8-ounce) can pineapple chunks, drained, juice reserved
1/4 cup dried cranberries
1/4 cup raisins
1 teaspoon cornstarch
12 maraschino cherries

Preheat the oven to warm and preheat a nonstick skillet over medium-low heat. Cook the ham slices, a few at a time, until they are lightly browned. Transfer them to a serving platter, cover, and place in the warm oven.

Pour the peach nectar into the skillet, scraping with a rubber spatula or wooden spoon to loosen brown bits from the bottom. Stir in the brown sugar, molasses, cloves, cinnamon, apricots, pineapple chunks, cranberries, and raisins. Reduce the heat to low and cook, stirring occasionally, until the mixture is bubbly and the dried fruit softens, about 10 minutes.

Place the cornstarch in a small bowl and whisk in 1 tablespoon of the reserved pineapple juice to form a slurry. Stir the cornstarch mixture into the fruit mixture, along with the cherries, and cook several minutes until the sauce thickens. To serve, spoon some of the fruit and sauce over the ham and pour the remainder into a serving bowl.

Yield: 8 to 10 servings

---

gyulai hungarian sausage and potatoes

Gyulai (pronounced July-e) sausage is fairly spicy, and when sautéed with potatoes, sweet onion, and garlic, it's quite savory, particularly on a chilly night. If you are unable to find Hungarian sausage in your local market, select another spicy sausage for similar results.

Ingredients:
5 small to medium red potatoes, scrubbed
1 tablespoon olive oil
1/2 cup chopped sweet onion
2 large cloves garlic, peeled and chopped
1 pound Gyulai Hungarian sausage, sliced 1/2 inch thick
Coarse salt and freshly ground black pepper, to taste

Slice the potatoes into quarters, place them in a medium saucepan with enough water to cover them, cover the pan, and bring the water to a boil over high heat. Reduce the heat to medium-low and cook 10 minutes, or until the potatoes are knife tender; drain.

Preheat a large cast-iron skillet over medium heat, add olive oil, and swirl to coat the bottom of the pan. Add the onion and garlic, and sauté 3 minutes until the onions are softened. Add the potatoes and sausage, reduce the heat to medium-low, and cook 15 minutes, stirring occasionally, until the potatoes are lightly browned. Season the dish with salt and pepper.

Yield: 4 to 6 servings

lamb chops with red currant mint sauce

If you've always wanted to cook like a chef, this is the recipe for you. Sautéed lamb chops glisten with a rich, meaty wine sauce, savory enough to have come from a restaurant kitchen, but easy enough that you can master this recipe in your own kitchen—and on a busy night at that! The secret is rich pan juices, fresh garlic, red wine, beef broth, and red currant jelly. Garnished with fresh mint, this dish is worthy of your family or your most important guests.

Ingredients:
1 tablespoon olive oil
2 to 4 lamb shoulder blade chops, or 4 to 8 loin chops
Coarse salt and freshly ground black pepper, to taste
2 large cloves garlic, peeled and minced
1/4 cup dry red wine
1/4 cup beef stock or broth
4 tablespoons red currant jelly
2 tablespoons fresh mint, cut into julienne
Mint leaves, for garnish

Preheat a large cast-iron skillet over medium heat and add the olive oil, swirling to coat the bottom of the pan. Season the lamb chops on both sides with salt and pepper, and cook them 3 to 4 minutes on each side, or until the meat is brown and the inside is rare. Cook the meat 2 minutes more on each side, remove it from the pan, and cover it to keep it warm.

Add the garlic and sauté 1 minute until it is soft. Deglaze the pan with wine and beef stock, stirring with a spatula or wooden spoon to loosen brown bits from the bottom of the pan. Add the jelly, stir until it has melted and the sauce begins to thicken, and reduce the heat to low.

Return the lamb chops to the pan, cover, and cook 2 to 3 minutes, until the meat is medium-rare. Sprinkle the meat with mint. To serve, transfer the meat to a platter, spoon the sauce over the meat, and garnish the platter with sprigs of fresh mint.

Yield: 2 to 4 servings

Cook's Tip: Lamb loin chops can be rather pricey for everyday meals. Shoulder blade chops have delicious lamb flavor without the loin chops' high price tag. Ask for them at your local supermarket or butcher shop.

---

lamb chops with dried plums and shiraz reduction

The title of this lamb chop recipe may sound complicated, but it truly is quick and easy to prepare. Lamb chops are browned on both sides in a skillet and popped in the oven for 10 minutes to finish cooking. Add a few ingredients to the skillet to make a sauce that tastes divine, and by the time the chops are ready, the sauce is too. You'll have an elegant dinner in less than 30 minutes.

Ingredients:
12 (1-inch-thick) lamb chops
Coarse salt and freshly ground black pepper, to taste
2 tablespoons fresh rosemary, chopped
1 tablespoon olive oil
1/2 cup Shiraz or Syrah wine
3/4 cup beef stock or broth
1 1/2 cups pitted dried plums
2 tablespoons cold unsalted butter
2 tablespoons flour
Sprigs of rosemary for garnish, if desired

Preheat the oven to 400°F and preheat a large skillet over medium heat. Season both sides of the lamb chops with salt, pepper, and rosemary. Pour the olive oil into the hot skillet, swirl to coat the bottom of the pan, and add half of the meat. Cook 4 to 5 minutes until the chops are brown, turn the meat over, and cook 3 to 4 minutes more to brown the other side.

27

Transfer the meat to a roasting pan, sear the remaining chops, and transfer them to the roasting pan. Roast the chops in a preheated oven 5 to 10 minutes, or until the meat is medium-rare. While the meat roasts, prepare the sauce.

Pour any accumulated fat from the skillet and deglaze the pan with the wine and beef stock, scraping up brown bits from the bottom of the pan with a rubber spatula or wooden spoon. Bring the mixture to a low boil, add dried plums, and cook 5 to 8 minutes, stirring occasionally, until the liquid is reduced by half. Season the sauce to taste with salt and pepper and reduce the heat to low.

Remove the skillet from the heat. Slice the butter into 4 pieces and dredge the pieces in flour until they are well coated. Stir the butter, one piece at a time, into the sauce until the butter is melted and the sauce is smooth. Remove the lamb chops from the oven, transfer them to a serving platter, and spoon the sauce over the meat. Garnish the platter with rosemary sprigs, if desired.

Yield: 6 servings

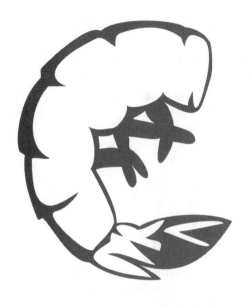

seafood

sautéed garlic shrimp spaghettini

Nothing cooks faster than shrimp sautéed, and when you add a good quality olive oil, lots of fresh garlic, and a bit of white wine and Parmesan cheese to the pan, your shrimp turn into a feast. Here, I've served succulent shrimp in white wine sauce over thin spaghetti called spaghettini. Just remember to save some of the water the pasta is cooked in for the sauce. Add candlelight and soft music, and dinner is ready.

Ingredients:
1/2 pound spaghettini or angel hair pasta,
  cooked according to package directions
1/4 to 1/2 cup reserved pasta water
1 tablespoon olive oil
1 tablespoon unsalted butter, optional
1/2 pound raw shrimp, peeled and deveined, tails removed
2 to 3 large cloves garlic, peeled and minced
1/4 cup seafood or vegetable broth
2 tablespoons white wine
2 tablespoon fresh parsley, chopped
1/4 cup Parmesan cheese, grated, plus additional for garnish

Drain the pasta, reserving 1/2 cup cooking water. Set the pasta aside and keep it warm.

Preheat a large skillet over medium heat, add the olive oil and butter, and swirl to melt the butter and coat the bottom of the pan. Add the shrimp and garlic, and cook, stirring constantly, about 3 minutes, or until the shrimp turn bright pink and the garlic is softened.

Deglaze the pan with seafood broth and white wine, stirring to loosen any bits of shrimp or garlic that are stuck to the bottom of the pan. Add 1/4 cup of the reserved pasta water, stir in the cooked pasta, and season it with salt and pepper.

Reduce the heat to low and add the parsley and Parmesan cheese, tossing to combine well. Add additional reserved pasta water if the pasta seems too dry. To serve, transfer the pasta to a large platter or pasta bowl and garnish it with additional grated Parmesan.

Yield: 4 servings

grilled skewered cajun shrimp

Talk about good! Cajun spices add a zesty flavor to this easy, fun recipe. When you're short on time, fire up the grill, thread shrimp onto metal skewers, and baste them with a Cajun-inspired butter sauce as they cook. What could be easier or more delicious!

Ingredients:
1/2 cup unsalted butter
1 small lemon or 1/2 of a large lemon, juiced
2 large cloves garlic, peeled and minced
3 drops Worcestershire sauce
1/2 teaspoon Cajun-style seasoning
1/8 teaspoon cayenne pepper
2 pounds large raw shrimp (16–20 count),
    peeled and deveined
4 metal skewers
Lemon wedges, for garnish
Sprigs of fresh Italian parsley, for garnish

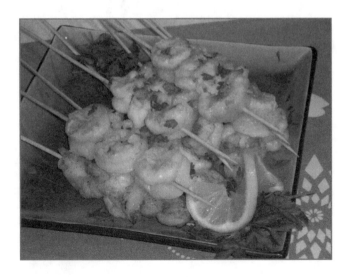

Preheat the grill to medium heat. In a small saucepan, melt the butter over medium-low heat and stir in the lemon juice, garlic, Worcestershire sauce, Cajun seasoning, and cayenne pepper. Reduce the heat to low and cook 3 to 4 minutes, stirring occasionally.

Thread 4 to 5 shrimp onto each skewer and place them on the grill. Baste the shrimp with the Cajun butter sauce and cook 2 minutes. Turn them over, baste with more of the sauce, and cook 2 to 3 minutes more, or until the shrimp are pink and tender. Take care not to overcook them.

To serve, transfer the skewered shrimp to a platter and garnish with wedges of lemon and sprigs of fresh parsley.

Yield: 4 servings

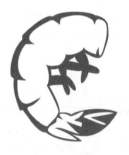

sautéed sea scallops

Fast meals don't have to look like fast food, as this recipe for sautéed sea scallops proves. Scallops taste best when they're cooked for a few short minutes to preserve their tenderness. Browning them lightly in the pan creates the basis for a delicate white wine sauce and results in an elegant dish after only minutes of preparation. Add a green vegetable, a glass of wine, and you're on your way to a relaxing evening.

Ingredients:
1 tablespoon olive oil
10 sea scallops, rinsed and dried on paper towels
1/4 cup dry white wine
1 lemon wedge
Coarse salt and freshly ground black pepper, to taste

Preheat a skillet over medium heat, add the olive oil, and swirl to coat the bottom of the pan. Add the scallops and sauté them 4 to 5 minutes, without stirring, until the bottoms are golden brown. Turn them over and sauté 3 to 4 minutes more until they brown on the bottom and are firm to the touch.

Transfer the scallops to a platter and cover them to keep them warm. Deglaze the pan with wine, stirring to loosen any brown bits, and cook until the liquid is reduced by half. Add a squeeze of lemon juice and season the sauce with salt and pepper. Pour the sauce over the scallops and serve.

Yield: 2 servings

seafood stew en papillote

Wild-caught halibut, black mussels, and sea scallops are steamed together in a parchment paper packet with fresh lemongrass, a bay leaf, and a splash of white wine. When the packet emerges from the oven 30 minutes later, you have a picture-perfect seafood stew for two requiring virtually no cleanup. Now, that's music to my ears!

Ingredients:
1 (18-inch) length parchment paper
2/3 pound wild-caught halibut steak
2 extra-large sea scallops
1/4 pound black mussels
Coarse salt and freshly ground black pepper, to taste
1/8 teaspoon paprika
1 stick lemongrass, peeled and cut into 6-inch lengths
1 bay leaf
1 tablespoon fresh parsley, chopped
2 tablespoons dry white wine

Preheat the oven to 350°F. Spread the parchment paper on a roasting pan or cookie sheet. Center the halibut in the paper and surround it with scallops and mussels. Sprinkle the seafood with salt, pepper, and paprika, and arrange lengths of lemongrass and the bay leaf on top of the fish. Sprinkle with parsley and wine.

Gather up the edges of the parchment paper, fold them down twice, and twist the ends securely to seal in the fish. Bake the packet 30 minutes, or until the fish is flaky and the mussels have opened. Discard any unopened mussels.

Transfer the parchment packet to a large serving platter, unfold, and serve.

Yield: 2 servings

wild-caught alaskan cod fillet en papillote

Cooking fish in parchment paper really reduces the mess and ensures a tender, flaky fish. Here, I've added broccoli florets, capers, sliced green onions, and lemon slices in the parchment packet for a flavorful meal that looks gorgeous on the platter.

Ingredients:
1 large sheet parchment paper
1 1/4 pounds wild-caught Alaskan cod fillet, rinsed and dried
Coarse salt and freshly ground black pepper, to taste
3 to 4 thin lemon slices
1/8 teaspoon paprika
1 tablespoon capers, rinsed and drained
1 green onion, white and green parts, sliced
1 sprig fresh parsley, chopped
1 1/2 cups broccoli florets

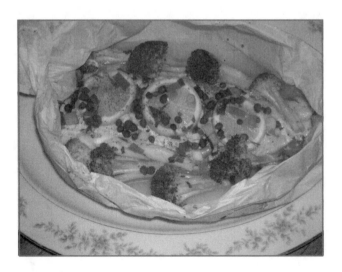

Preheat the oven to 350°F. Spread the parchment paper on a large baking pan or cookie sheet and place the fish in the center of the paper. Season the fish with salt and pepper, arrange lemon slices on the top, and sprinkle with paprika, capers, sliced onion, and parsley. Arrange the broccoli florets along both sides of the fish.

Gather up the edges of the parchment paper, fold them down twice, and twist the ends securely to seal in the fish. Bake the packet 25 minutes, or until the fish is flaky and the broccoli is tender when pierced with a sharp knife.

Transfer the parchment packet to a large serving platter, unfold, and serve.

Yield: 2 to 3 servings

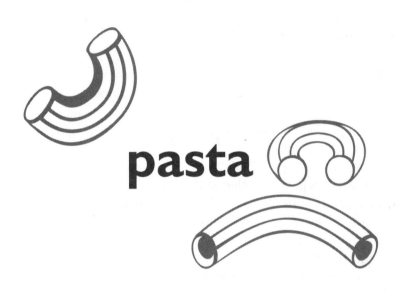

pasta

creamy spinach fettuccine with mushrooms and prosciutto

The day I created this recipe, I shared a goodly portion with our Colorado friends, the Werts. It happened to be one of those busy days full of after-school activities for their sons, and Debbie told me my phone message inquiring whether she would like pasta, minestrone, and pizza for dinner was a dream come true. In truth, with just a few ingredients, Debbie could have whipped up this recipe herself in less than 30 minutes, but it was fun playing her fairy godmother that day.

Ingredients:
1/2 pound spinach fettuccine, cooked according
   to package directions
1/4 cup reserved pasta water
2 tablespoon olive oil
2 cups mushrooms, sliced
3 large cloves garlic, peeled and minced
2 ounces prosciutto, cut into 1/2-inch pieces
1/4 cup dry white wine
1/2 cup heavy cream
1/4 teaspoon coarse salt
Freshly ground black pepper, to taste
1/4 cup Pecorino Romano cheese,
   grated, plus additional for garnish

Drain the pasta, reserving 1/4 cup of the cooking water. Set the pasta aside and keep it warm.

Preheat a large skillet over medium heat, add the olive oil, and swirl to coat the bottom of the pan. Add the mushrooms, sauté 1 minute, and add the garlic and prosciutto. Sauté 2 minutes more, stirring constantly.

Stir in the white wine, reserved pasta water, heavy cream, salt, and pepper. Raise the heat to medium-high, bring the mixture to a boil, and cook, stirring frequently, 3 minutes, until the liquid is reduced by one-fourth.

Remove the skillet from the heat, add the cooked pasta and Romano cheese, and stir gently to mix. Transfer the pasta to a large serving bowl, garnish it with additional grated cheese, and serve.

Yield: 4 servings

---

cellentani and italian sausage pasticcio

Pasticcio is an Italian oven-baked, layered pasta dish, similar to lasagna but made with short, macaroni-style pasta, like the corkscrew-shaped cellentani used in this version. Shells, penne, ziti, and farfalle also work well in pasticcio. In my version, I layer fresh basil, Romano cheese, ricotta, and mozzarella with my spicy Italian Sausage Pasta Sauce (see page 41). To personalize your pasticcio, add sliced mushrooms, eggplant, zucchini, or your favorite lasagna fillings.

Ingredients:
1 (15-ounce) carton part-skim ricotta cheese
1 egg
1 recipe Italian Sausage Pasta Sauce
1 (16-ounce) package cellentani or other
    macaroni-style pasta, cooked al dente
1 cup Pecorino Romano cheese, grated
10 fresh basil leaves, torn
3/4 cup mozzarella, grated

Preheat the oven to 375°F. In a small bowl, stir together the ricotta cheese and egg until the mixture is creamy; set aside.

Spread 3/4 cup of Italian Sausage Pasta Sauce in the bottom of a 10-cup casserole dish. Top with one-third of the cooked pasta, 1 cup of the sauce, half of the ricotta cheese mixture, half of the

Romano cheese, and half of the basil. Add half of the remaining pasta, 1 cup of the sauce, the remaining ricotta cheese mixture, the remaining Romano cheese, half of the mozzarella, and the remaining basil.

For the top layer, spread the remaining pasta, top with the remaining sauce, and sprinkle on the remaining mozzarella. Cover and bake the casserole 30 minutes, or until the dish is hot and bubbly. Remove the casserole from the oven, set it aside for 10 minutes to allow it to set, and serve.

Yield: 8 servings

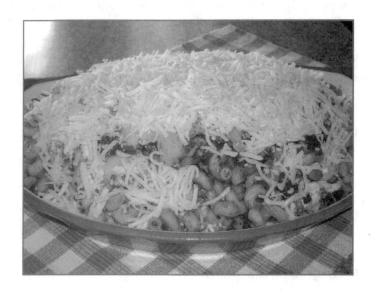

italian sausage pasta sauce

My husband, Randy, loves spicy foods that give a little kick in the back of the throat, and so he really enjoys this flavorful sauce. The recipe includes ingredients from the pantry or spice cabinet, plus a few fresh items I like to keep on hand, so it's easy to stir up a batch of sauce at a moment's notice. Serve the sauce over any pasta, or for a real taste treat on the weekend, use it to create pasticcio, a traditional Italian layered pasta dish. You'll find my own flavor-packed version of pasticcio on page 39.

Ingredients:
1 tablespoon olive oil
1 pound Italian sausage
5 large cloves garlic, chopped
1 (15-ounce) can petite diced tomatoes
1 (15-ounce) can tomato sauce
1 teaspoon dried basil
1/4 teaspoon red pepper flakes
1 dash sugar
Freshly ground black pepper, to taste

Preheat a large skillet or saucepan over medium heat, add the olive oil, and swirl to coat the bottom of the pan. Add the sausage to the pan, breaking it into pieces with a wooden spoon as it cooks, and sauté until it is no longer pink inside, about 6 to 8 minutes.

Drain any fat that has accumulated in the bottom of the skillet, reduce the heat to medium-low, and add the garlic. Sauté the garlic 1 minute until it is soft and fragrant. Stir in the diced tomatoes, tomato sauce, dried basil, red pepper flakes, sugar, and pepper.

Reduce the heat to low, cover the skillet with the lid off center, and cook the sauce 15 to 30 minutes, stirring occasionally.

Yield: 8 servings

fusilli with artichokes and asparagus

I love pasta salads as both side dishes and as main courses. This salad is particularly refreshing on a spring or summer day, and if you store fusilli pasta, canned artichokes, and kalamata olives in your pantry, you can have the meal on the table in no time.

Ingredients:
1 pound asparagus, rinsed and trimmed
1 pound fusilli pasta, cooked al dente
1 (14-ounce) can quartered artichokes, drained
1 1/2 cups cherry tomatoes, rinsed and halved
1/2 cup pitted kalamata olives
1/3 cup chopped red onion
1/3 tablespoon fresh basil, chopped
Coarse salt and freshly ground black pepper, to taste
1/2 cup olive oil
2 tablespoons balsamic vinegar
1/2 teaspoon Dijon mustard
2 large cloves garlic, minced
Fresh basil leaves, for garnish
Parmesan cheese, grated, for garnish

Slice the asparagus at an angle into 2-inch lengths. Place the asparagus pieces in a shallow saucepan, add water to a depth of 1/4 inch, cover, and bring to a boil. Reduce the heat to low and cook 1 minute, until the vegetables are crisp-tender. Immediately transfer the blanched asparagus to a large bowl of ice water to stop the cooking process, drain, and set aside.

In a large pasta bowl, combine the fusilli, artichokes, cherry tomatoes, kalamata olives, red onion, fresh basil, and asparagus. Season the pasta with salt and pepper.

In a small bowl, whisk together olive oil, balsamic vinegar, Dijon mustard, garlic, salt, and pepper until mixed. Pour the vinaigrette over the pasta and toss well. Garnish the dish with a large sprig of fresh basil and Parmesan cheese, if desired. Serve pasta warm or chilled.

Yield: 8 servings

green and white farfalle with sweet peas and sage derby cheese

This recipe was inspired by one that my friend and chef, Mick Weisberg, made on my Texas television cooking show a couple of years ago. In my version, I incorporated fresh garden peas I purchased at the Dillon, Colorado, farmers market and sage Derby cheese, which is variegated green and white and has a lovely fresh sage fragrance. Mick uses avocados that are so ripe they become a sauce when mixed with the pasta. My version uses soft avocados that still hold their shape and depends more upon the garlic, olive oil, and cheese for the overall flavor. I think you'll absolutely love the end result.

Ingredients:
1/2 pound farfalle pasta, cooked according
   to package directions
1/4 cup reserved pasta water
2 tablespoons olive oil, divided
2 large cloves garlic, peeled and minced
1 cup fresh sweet peas, cooked until tender,
   or 1 cup frozen peas, thawed
1 very ripe avocado
1/2 cup sage Derby cheese, grated
Coarse salt and freshly ground black pepper, to taste

Drain the pasta, reserving 1/4 cup of the cooking water. Set the pasta aside and keep it warm. Add 1 tablespoon of the olive oil to the pasta pot, swirl to coat the bottom of the pan, and add the garlic. Sauté the garlic 1 minute, add the peas, and cook 1 minute more. Remove the pan from the heat and stir in the pasta.

Slice the avocado in half, remove the pit, and using a knife, slice the pulp into 1/4-inch cubes. With a large spoon, scoop out the pulp from the shell and stir it into the pasta. Add the cheese, season with salt and pepper, and stir gently to mix.

Yield: 4 to 6 servings

italian lasagna

This classic dish is sheer comfort food—perfect after a hectic day at the office, keeping up with kids' schedules, or weekend enjoyment. No-boil lasagna noodles reduce the preparation time and mess, making this family favorite possible even on the busiest days. Just combine the sauce ingredients, layer the sauce with pasta and cheese, and pop the dish in the oven. Choose part-skim or no-fat ricotta for great flavor without the fat. Leftovers are just as tasty the next day and freeze beautifully for another meal.

Ingredients:
2 tablespoons olive oil
1 cup chopped onion
4 large cloves garlic, minced
1 (28-ounce) can petite diced tomatoes
1 (15-ounce) can tomato sauce
3 tablespoons tomato paste
1 1/2 tablespoons dried oregano
1 teaspoon dried basil
1 teaspoon anise seed, crushed with a mortar and pestle
Freshly ground black pepper, to taste
1 egg, beaten
1 (15-ounce) container part-skim or no-fat ricotta cheese
1 (9-ounce) package no-boil lasagna pasta
3 cups shredded mozzarella cheese
2/3 cup Pecorino Romano or Parmesan, grated

To make the sauce, in a large saucepan over medium heat, add the olive oil, and swirl to coat the bottom of the pan. Add the onion and sauté 3 minutes until it is soft; add the garlic and cook 1 minute more. Stir in the diced tomatoes, tomato sauce, tomato paste, oregano, basil, anise seed, and black pepper. Cook until the sauce starts to boil, then reduce heat to low and cook 10 minutes more.

Preheat the oven to 375°F. In a small bowl, stir together the egg and ricotta cheese until the ricotta is light and fluffy; set aside.

Pour 1 1/3 cups of the sauce into the bottom of a 9x13-inch baking pan and spread it across the bottom with a spatula. Layer 4 lasagna noodles, 1 cup of the sauce, one-third of the ricotta mixture, and 1 cup shredded mozzarella. Repeat process once, then layer 4 lasagna noodles, 1 cup sauce, remaining ricotta mixture, and the grated Pecorino Romano. Top with remaining lasagna noodles, sauce, and mozzarella, for a total of 4 layers. Cover the pan tightly with foil.

Bake the lasagna 40 to 50 minutes, or until it is hot and bubbly. Remove the dish from the oven, set aside 10 minutes to allow it to set, and serve.

Yield: 8 servings

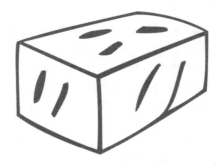

mostaccioli and spinach with pecorino romano

This is an uncomplicated recipe for simple food, but its subtle flavors blend to form a lasting impression. For a family meal or romantic candlelit dinner for two, this pasta dish is utterly sublime.

Ingredients:
1 (12-ounce) package Mostaccioli pasta,
   cooked according to package directions
1/4 to 1/2 cup reserved pasta water
2 tablespoons olive oil
2 tablespoons shallots, minced
3 large cloves garlic, minced
1/3 cup dry white wine
1/4 cup chicken or vegetable broth
Coarse salt and freshly ground black pepper, to taste
2 cups fresh baby spinach, washed, dried, and stemmed
1/3 cup Pecorino Romano cheese, shaved

When the pasta is cooked al dente, drain it, reserving 1/2 cup of the pasta water. Set the pasta aside and keep it warm.

Heat a medium skillet over medium-low heat, add the olive oil, and swirl to coat the bottom of the pan. Sauté the shallots 2 to 3 minutes until they turn translucent, add the garlic, and cook 1 minute more.

Deglaze the pan with white wine, chicken broth, and 1/4 cup of the reserved pasta water. Raise the heat to medium, bring the mixture to a boil, and cook several minutes until the sauce is reduced by one-third. Season the sauce with salt and pepper.

Stir in the fresh spinach and cook just until it begins to wilt, about 1 minute. Add additional reserved pasta water if the liquid evaporates too quickly. Spoon the mixture over the warm pasta and top with shavings of Pecorino Romano.

Yield: 4 servings

penne pomodoro with roasted bell pepper sauce

I'm wild about this pasta recipe. Roasted red bell peppers add an extra dimension to this classic Italian dish, without complicating the recipe or overwhelming the fresh flavor of the tomato sauce. You'll find jars of marinated roasted red bell peppers in most supermarkets, usually in the aisle with the olives. Try them on burgers, in salads and pasta, and in Southwest-inspired dishes.

Ingredients:
1 (16-ounce) package penne pasta,
   cooked according to package directions
1/4 to 1/2 cup reserved pasta water
3 tablespoons olive oil
5 large cloves garlic, peeled and minced
3 ripe Roma tomatoes, chopped
1 (15-ounce) can petite diced tomatoes
1/2 cup marinated roasted red peppers,
   drained and chopped
1 tablespoon dried basil
1/2 teaspoon coarse salt
Freshly ground black pepper, to taste
3 to 4 large leaves fresh basil, cut into julienne
Parmigiano Reggiano, grated, for garnish

Drain the cooked pasta, reserving 1/2 cup of the pasta water for use in the sauce. Set the pasta aside and keep it warm.

Preheat a large skillet over medium heat, add the olive oil, and swirl to coat the bottom of the pan. Add the garlic and sauté 1 minute, stirring constantly, then add the Roma tomatoes and cook them 3 minutes, until they soften.

Stir in the canned tomatoes, 1/4 cup of the reserved pasta water, roasted peppers, dried basil, salt, and pepper. Reduce the heat to medium-low and cook the sauce 8 to 10 minutes, stirring occasionally.

Just before serving, add the cooked pasta, the fresh basil, and, if the mixture seems too dry, a little of the reserved pasta water to the sauce. Check the seasonings, transfer the pasta to a large serving bowl, and garnish with grated Parmigiano Reggiano.

Yield: 6 servings

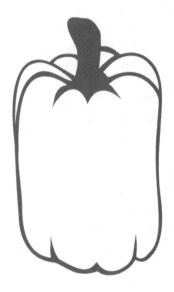

southwest orzo with roasted red pepper pesto

If you love Southwest-inspired flavors, you'll love the pesto featured in this pasta dish. Use it to flavor pasta as I've done here, or as a garnish for meats, poultry, and fish. The pesto takes just a few minutes to prepare, thanks to pre-roasted peppers you'll find in jars in the supermarket aisle with the olives. Just place the ingredients in a food processor, give it a quick whirl, and the pesto is ready.

Ingredients:
1/2 cup roasted red sweet peppers
1/3 cup fresh basil leaves
1/4 cup pine nuts
1 large or 2 small cloves fresh garlic, peeled
1/2 teaspoon coarse salt
Freshly ground black pepper, to taste
1/3 cup olive oil
1/2 pound Southwest or plain orzo pasta,
    cooked according to package directions

In the bowl of a food processor, combine the roasted peppers, basil, pine nuts, garlic, salt, and pepper. Process until the mixture is well blended. With the processor on low speed, slowly pour the oil in a steady stream until the mixture is smooth and well blended; set aside.

When the pasta is done, stir in half of the pesto and transfer it to a serving bowl. Spoon the remaining pesto into a serving bowl and pass it along with the pasta.

Yield: 4 to 6 servings

three-cheese macaroni

While this recipe won't win any awards in the "low-fat" category, an occasional splurge can be good for the spirit, especially when you crave comfort food. For quick meals, purchase grated cheese instead of grating your own, and serve this creamy dish straight from the pot, but if you love crispy edges and a crunchy bread crumb topping, I highly recommend transferring the macaroni and cheese to a casserole dish and popping it into the oven for a few minutes while setting the table and preparing a vegetable or salad. Either way, my judges give this recipe a "10" for family favorite.

Ingredients:
1 (16-ounce) package elbow macaroni,
   cooked according to package directions
1/3 cup butter
1 1/4 cups half-and-half
2 cups aged Provolone cheese, grated
2 cups medium cheddar cheese, grated
1 1/2 cups Monterey Jack cheese, grated
Coarse salt and freshly ground black pepper, to taste
1/4 cup plain or seasoned bread crumbs (optional)

Drain the cooked pasta and cover it to keep it warm. In the pasta pot, melt the butter over medium-low heat, add the half-and-half, and bring the mixture to a boil. Return the macaroni to the pot and stir.

Add the Provolone, cheddar, and Monterey Jack cheeses and stir gently until they have melted. Season with salt and pepper and stir to mix.

To serve, spoon macaroni and cheese directly from the pot, or preheat the oven to 350°F and grease a casserole dish. Transfer the pasta to the casserole dish, sprinkle the top with bread crumbs, and bake 20 to 30 minutes until it is hot and bubbly.

Yield: 6 to 8 servings

tortellini, garlic, and mushrooms

This pasta recipe is simple but so satisfying. The combination of little pillows of pasta, fragrant garlic, tasty mushrooms, and freshly grated Pecorino Romano cheese is perfect at the end of a stressful day when you need a nutritious meal in a *hurry*. Add a salad and perhaps a glass of wine, and you're all set.

Ingredients:
1 (7-ounce) package tortellini, cooked according
   to package directions
1/2 cup reserved pasta water
2 tablespoons olive oil
1/2 pound sliced mushrooms
3 large cloves garlic
3 tablespoons chicken or vegetable stock or broth
1/3 cup Pecorino Romano cheese, grated,
   plus more for garnish
Coarse salt and freshly ground black pepper, to taste
2 sprigs fresh parsley, chopped

When the pasta is cooked al dente, drain, reserving 1/2 cup of the pasta water. Set the pasta aside and cover it to keep it warm.

Heat a large skillet over medium-low heat, add the olive oil, and swirl to coat the bottom of the pan. Add the mushrooms and sauté 2 minutes, stirring frequently. Add the garlic and sauté 1 minute more.

Stir in the cooked tortellini, reserved pasta water, chicken stock, and 1/3 cup of the Romano cheese. Cook, stirring often, until most of the liquid is absorbed and the pasta is fragrant, about 5 minutes.

Season the pasta with salt and pepper, sprinkle it with parsley, and stir gently. Transfer it to a serving bowl and garnish with additional grated cheese.

Yield: 2 to 3 servings

whole-wheat pasta with chicken and tomato-leek sauce

Transform any night into Italian night with a red-checked table-cloth, candlelight, and this whole-wheat pasta dish with slightly spicy red sauce. Follow the recipe and quickly sauté tender strips of boneless chicken breast, or prepare a vegetarian version by omitting the chicken. Either way, that's Italian!

Ingredients:
3 tablespoons olive oil, divided
2 pounds skinless, boneless chicken breast,
    cut into thin strips
2 leeks, white part only, rinsed and diced
2 large cloves garlic, peeled and minced
1/4 cup dry white wine
1/2 cup chicken stock
1 (28-ounce) can diced tomatoes
1 teaspoon dried oregano
1/2 teaspoon red pepper flakes
1/4 teaspoon sugar
Coarse salt and freshly ground black pepper, to taste
1 tablespoon chopped Italian parsley
1 tablespoon chopped fresh oregano
1 pound whole-wheat pasta, cooked according
    to package directions

Preheat a large skillet over medium heat, add 2 tablespoons of the olive oil, and swirl to coat the bottom of the pan. Add half of the chicken strips, cook 1 to 2 minutes without stirring until one side is brown, and turn them over to brown the other side. Transfer the cooked chicken to a bowl. Cook the remaining chicken strips, transfer them to the bowl, and keep them warm.

Pour the remaining olive oil into the skillet, add the leeks and garlic, and cook 1 to 2 minutes until the leeks are soft. Stir in the wine, chicken stock, tomatoes, dried oregano, red pepper flakes, sugar, salt, and pepper. Reduce the heat to medium-low and cook the sauce 5 minutes, stirring frequently.

Reduce the heat to low, stir in the cooked chicken, parsley, and fresh oregano, and cook 10 minutes more. Serve over whole-wheat pasta.

Yield: 6 servings

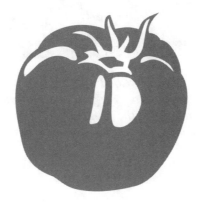

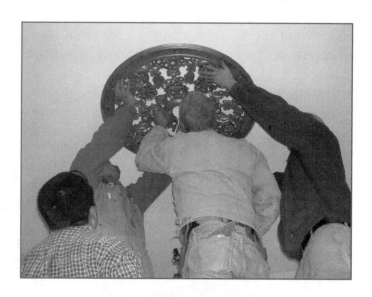

Good As Gold:
Our crew carefully replaces a large gold plaster medallion that anchors an antique crystal chandalier in the living room. The medallion and chandalier originally graced a popular Denver, Colorado restaurant in the 1870's.

pizza

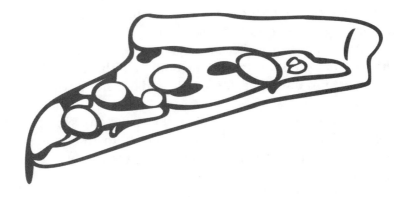

caramelized sweet onion, spinach, and feta pizzas

This is one of my most popular recipes for casual gatherings and light suppers. I start with packaged pizza crusts and transform them into gourmet fare with caramelized sweet onions, sautéed fresh spinach, canned artichokes, and feta cheese. The combination of the chewy dough and still-crunchy onions and the sweet and tangy flavors on the fresh-from-the-oven pizza crust create a wonderfully deluxe dish. And best of all, you can assemble the pizzas hours ahead of time and pop them in the oven just before serving.

Ingredients:
2 (8-inch) pizza crusts
4 tablespoons olive oil, divided
Coarse salt, to taste
3 cups fresh spinach leaves, rinsed and dried
1 large sweet onion, peeled and sliced
1 (14-ounce) can artichoke hearts, drained and quartered
2 ounces crumbled feta cheese

Preheat the oven to 425°F. Place the pizza crusts on a large cookie sheet, brush the tops with 1 tablespoon of the olive oil, sprinkle lightly with salt, and set aside.

Preheat a large skillet over medium heat, add 1 tablespoon of the olive oil, and swirl to coat the bottom of the pan. Add the spinach, sauté just until it begins to wilt, and transfer it with tongs onto the pizza crusts.

Add the remaining olive oil to the skillet and swirl to coat the bottom of the pan. Add onion and sauté 10 to 15 minutes, stirring occasionally, until it is golden brown. Layer the onion on top of the spinach.

Arrange artichokes on top of the onions and sprinkle with feta cheese. Bake 10 to 12 minutes until the pizzas are hot. Slice each pizza into 6 pieces and serve.

Yield: 2 dinner servings or 4 appetizer servings

Cook's Tip: Caramelizing onions works best with sweet onions because they have more natural sugar in them than storage onions. Avoid the temptation to stir the onions frequently until they begin to brown. If the onions tend to steam rather than brown, drain off excess onion juices, add 1 tablespoon butter (not margarine) to the pan, and raise the heat slightly.

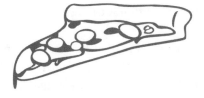

57

red onion, mushroom, and fresh mozzarella pizzas

Still-crunchy red onions, tender mushrooms, and creamy fresh mozzarella top these luscious pizzas. For a hot lunch, quick snack, or easy-does-it dinner, convenient packaged pizza crusts and every-day ingredients team up for a definite crowd pleaser.

Ingredients:
2 (8-inch) pizza crusts
2 tablespoons olive oil, divided
Coarse salt, to taste
2 cups mushrooms, sliced
1/2 cup red onion, chopped
2 tablespoons fresh parsley, chopped
4 ounces fresh mozzarella cheese
1/2 cup sliced black olives

Preheat the oven to 425°F. Place the pizza crusts on a large cookie sheet, brush the tops with 1 tablespoon of the olive oil, sprinkle lightly with salt, and set aside.

Preheat a large skillet over medium heat, add the remaining olive oil, and swirl to coat the bottom of the pan. Add mushrooms and onion, sauté 2 minutes until the onions are crisp-tender, and sprinkle with parsley. Stir to mix and set aside.

Slice mozzarella and arrange it on top of the pizza crusts. Spoon the mushroom mixture over the cheese and sprinkle it with black olives. Bake 10 to 12 minutes until the pizzas are hot. Slice each pizza into 6 pieces and serve.

Yield: 2 dinner servings or 4 appetizer servings

tomato basil pizzas

I served these mini pizzas to a friend in Colorado when she came over for a glass of wine one afternoon. It took me about 10 minutes to prepare them, and after they baked a few minutes in the oven, we were noshing on pizzas topped with gooey strings of melted mozzarella cheese, fresh garden tomatoes, green onions, and tangy Gorgonzola. Although I love making my own fragrant pizza dough, for quick and easy snacks or meals, packaged pizza crusts are the way to go. Add your favorite ingredients and you're on your way to great eating!

Ingredients:
2 (8-inch) pizza crusts
1 tablespoon olive oil
1/8 teaspoon coarse salt
1 cup mozzarella cheese, grated
2 green onions, white and green parts, sliced
1 to 2 ripe tomatoes, thinly sliced
Freshly ground black pepper
3 large leaves fresh basil, rolled and cut into julienne
1/3 cup Gorgonzola cheese, crumbled

Preheat the oven to 425°F. Place the pizza crusts on a large cookie sheet, brush the tops with olive oil, and sprinkle them with salt.

Top the pizza crusts with mozzarella cheese, green onions, and sliced tomato. Season them with freshly ground pepper and sprinkle with basil and crumbled Gorgonzola cheese.

Bake 10 to 12 minutes until the pizzas are hot and the mozzarella has melted. Slice each pizza into 6 pieces and serve.

Yield: 2 dinner servings or 4 appetizer servings

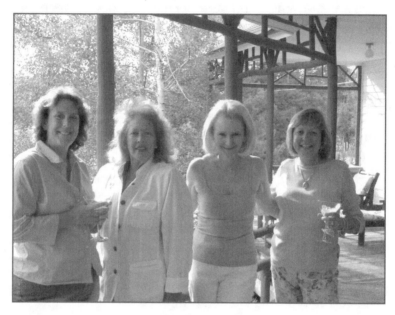

Party Girls:
*For our first summer porch party, all the ladies showed up wearing pink.
I didn't even send out a memo! With the old kitchen out of commission,
preparing the menu in my tiny condo kitchen and hauling it over in
the car made this first dinner gathering possible.*

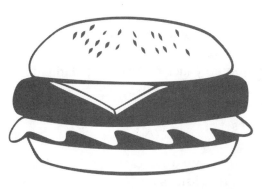

sandwiches

black bean burritos

Here's a quick, tasty recipe for fast meals or sheer enjoyment. Canned black beans, chopped onion, and cheese are rolled into flour tortillas and baked until they're hot, and served with prepared picante sauce. For those who love heat, sliced jalepeños garnish the top.

Ingredients:
4 (6-inch) flour tortillas
1 (15-ounce) can black beans, rinsed and drained
1/3 cup onion, chopped
1 1/2 cups cheddar or Monterey Jack cheese, grated, divided
1 1/4 cups prepared picante sauce or salsa
1 jalapeño, sliced
3/4 cup sliced black olives

Preheat the oven to 350°F. Spray a large casserole dish with nonstick cooking spray and set the dish aside.

In the center of a flour tortilla, spoon one-quarter of the black beans, one-quarter of the onion, and 1/4 cup of the cheese. Roll up the tortilla and transfer it to a casserole dish with the seam facing down. Repeat the process with the remaining tortillas and fillings, being sure to reserve 1/2 cup cheese for the topping.

Pour the picante sauce over the burritos and top with the remaining cheese, jalapeño, and black olives. Cover the dish tightly with foil and bake 30 minutes, or until the burritos are hot and the cheese has melted.

Yield: 4 burritos

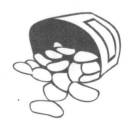

chicken club quesadilla

This quesadilla makes a tasty lunch or appetizer or a quick and easy dinner, and it's a great way to use leftover cooked chicken. I substitute turkey bacon for the regular bacon, to get the same flavor without all the fat.

Ingredients:
1 grilled chicken breast half, sliced
1 1/2 cups cheddar cheese, grated
1/4 cup crisp turkey bacon, crumbled
1 large tomato, chopped
2 teaspoons fresh cilantro, chopped
4 8-inch flour tortillas
2 teaspoons olive oil
Pico de gallo or salsa, optional
Tortilla chips, optional

Preheat a large nonstick skillet over medium heat. Layer half of the chicken, 3/4 cup of the cheese, 2 tablespoons of the bacon, half of the tomato, and 1 teaspoon of the cilantro onto each of the 2 tortillas. Cover each quesadilla with one of the remaining 2 tortillas.

Pour the olive oil into the hot skillet and swirl it to coat the bottom of the pan. Cook each quesadilla 3 minutes, turn it over, and cook 1 to 2 minutes more, until the fillings are hot and the cheese is melted. Remove the quesadillas from the skillet and slice them into quarters. Serve with pico de gallo and tortilla chips, if desired.

Yield: 2 dinner servings or 8 appetizer servings.

deluxe grilled fontina sandwiches

This sandwich idea came during the final weeks of writing this book when I hadn't had time to go grocery shopping, and my husband, Randy, and I were in need of a quick lunch. I set out four slices of bread, thinly sliced some cheese, sautéed onion and bell peppers until the onions were golden, and created a wonderfully fragrant sandwich. It just goes to show that even when the refrigerator looks empty, the ingredients for a memorable meal may be just inside the next drawer.

Ingredients:
1 tablespoon olive oil
3 thick slices of onion
1/2 bell pepper, any color, sliced
4 slices of bread
6 slices Fontina, Monterey Jack, or Cheddar cheese
1 scant tablespoon butter

Preheat a large skillet over medium heat. Add the olive oil and swirl to coat the bottom of the pan. Add the onions and peppers, and sauté, stirring occasionally, until the onions are golden brown, about 10 minutes.

Arrange 3 cheese slices on each of two slices of bread and top with sautéed onions and peppers. Top with the remaining bread slices. Melt butter in the skillet and toast the sandwiches 3 to 4 minutes on each side until the bread is golden brown and the cheese has melted.

Slice the sandwiches in half and serve immediately.

Yield: 2 sandwiches

grilled chicken and veggie pockets with creamy mustard dressing

For a light, easy meal these sandwiches really hit the spot. Seasoned grilled chicken is tucked into pita pockets with crunchy bell peppers and golden sweet onions. As if that weren't scrumptious enough, I drizzle spicy yogurt mustard dressing over the top. Mmm, sensational!

Ingredients:
3/4 cup nonfat plain yogurt
3 tablespoons mayonnaise
1 tablespoon sweet onion, diced
2 teaspoons coarse-grain mustard
1 teaspoon freshly squeezed lemon juice
1/2 teaspoon cumin
1/4 teaspoon coarse salt
1/8 teaspoon cayenne pepper
Pinch of white pepper
4 drops Tabasco sauce
1 1/4 pounds chicken tenders
1 teaspoon garlic powder
1 teaspoon onion powder
1/2 teaspoon coarse salt
1/4 teaspoon freshly ground black pepper
1 tablespoon olive oil
1 large sweet onion, peeled and sliced
3 cloves garlic, peeled and diced
1 large green bell pepper, sliced
1 large red bell pepper, sliced
3/4 teaspoon cumin
8 pita pockets

In a medium bowl, stir together yogurt, mayonnaise, 1 tablespoon onion, mustard, lemon juice, cumin, 1/4 teaspoon of the salt, cayenne pepper, white pepper, and Tabasco. Cover and chill 30 minutes.

Preheat the grill to medium heat. Rinse the chicken tenders, pat them dry on paper towels, and set them aside. In a small bowl, stir together the garlic powder, onion powder, salt, and pepper. Season the chicken well with some of the mixture and set the remainder aside for use later.

Preheat a large skillet over medium heat, add the olive oil, and swirl to coat the bottom of the pan. Add the onions and sauté 10 to 15 minutes, stirring occasionally, until they turn golden brown. Add the garlic and bell peppers, and cook until the vegetables are crisptender. Season the vegetables with 1/2 teaspoon of the reserved seasoning mixture and stir well. Transfer the vegetables to a serving bowl and cover to keep them warm.

Grill the chicken tenders, slice them, and transfer them to a serving platter. Slice the pita bread in half and fill each pocket with grilled chicken and sautéed onion and peppers. Drizzle each with mustard sauce and serve.

Yield: 8 sandwiches

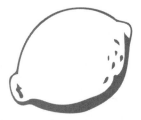

grilled hamburgers with gorgonzola and roasted peppers

Hamburgers can be a quick meal, but when they're grilled and garnished with gorgonzola cheese and roasted peppers, you may elect to serve them even when time isn't a limiting factor. I love the tangy flavor of Gorgonzola as it softens from the heat of the grill, and when it's paired with grilled beef and roasted peppers straight from a jar, this simple meal becomes sheer delight.

Ingredients:
4 hamburger patties
Coarse salt and freshly ground black pepper, to taste
1 (12-ounce) jar roasted red sweet peppers
4 ounces Gorgonzola cheese, sliced
4 wheat rolls

Preheat the outdoor grill. When the grill is hot, season the hamburger patties and place them on the grill. Cook 4 to 5 minutes depending on their thickness, turn them over, and cook until they are almost done, 4 to 5 minutes more.

Top the meat with strips of roasted pepper and slices of Gorgonzola cheese. Close the cover on the grill and cook 1 minute more, or until the cheese begins to soften and the meat is cooked to the desired degree of doneness.

Remove the meat from the grill and serve on toasted rolls. Garnish as desired.

Yield: 4 sandwiches

grilled veggie and pepper cheese paninis

You'll never miss the meat in this robust vegetarian sandwich. Crusty artisan bread is packed with slices of grilled zucchini, yellow squash, eggplant, and hot pepper cheese. Then it's briefly toasted on the grill or an electric panini press until the cheese is melted and the bread is scored and golden brown. Eating well can be such a tasteful experience!

Ingredients:
1 loaf focaccia or other flat artisan bread
1 cup olive oil, divided
3 zucchini, halved and thinly sliced lengthwise
3 yellow squash, sliced thinly at an angle
1 small eggplant, peeled and thinly sliced
8 ounces hot pepper cheese, sliced

Preheat the outdoor grill or electric panini press. Slice the bread into thick wedges and slice each wedge in half crosswise. Brush the cut sides with about 1/2 cup of the olive oil.

While the grill is preheating, brush the zucchini, yellow squash, and eggplant with about 3 tablespoons of the olive oil. When the grill is hot, cook the vegetables until they are soft and have nice grill marks, about 1 minute on each side.

Layer grilled vegetables and cheese on the lower half of each wedge of bread. Replace the top half and brush the outer surfaces with about 1/4 cup of the olive oil. Transfer paninis to the grill and place a large iron skillet or foil-covered brick on top of them to flatten them while they cook. When the bread is slightly toasted, flip the paninis over with a spatula and toast the other side.

If you are using an electric panini press, preheat and brush the press lightly with olive oil. Grill the vegetables and assemble the paninis as above. Transfer the paninis to the preheated press, lower the cover, and grill until the bread is lightly toasted and the cheese has melted.

Yield: 6 to 8 sandwiches

lamb and mushroom pitas with mint-yogurt dressing

For an easy meal that's high on flavor and fun, serve these tasty pita sandwiches. No need to stand in the take-out line for a fast meal, when the supermarket does most of the prep work. I use pre-cut lamb stew meat, so after a final quick trim, the meat is ready for the skillet. It's sautéed with garlic and mushrooms in a lovely beef broth, wine, and rosemary sauce, and then it's tucked into pita pockets and served with a mint-yogurt dressing that perfectly complements the lamb.

Ingredients:
1 cup plain yogurt
1 tablespoon fresh mint, chopped
1/2 teaspoon coarse salt, divided
1/8 teaspoon chili powder or paprika
1/8 teaspoon garlic powder
1/8 teaspoon onion powder
Freshly ground pepper mélange, to taste
1 tablespoon olive oil
1 pound lamb stew meat, trimmed of fat and cartilage
2 shallots, peeled and chopped
2 large cloves garlic, peeled and minced
1/2 pound mushrooms, sliced
1 tablespoon beef stock or broth
1 tablespoon dry red wine
1 teaspoon dried rosemary, crushed
Freshly ground black pepper, to taste
6 pita pockets

In a small bowl, stir together yogurt, mint, 1/4 teaspoon of the salt, chili powder, garlic powder, onion powder, and pepper mélange until it is smooth. Set aside.

Preheat a large skillet over medium heat, add the olive oil, and swirl to coat the bottom of the pan. Add the stew meat and shallots, and cook 2 minutes without stirring, until the meat starts to brown on the bottom. Add the garlic and mushrooms, stir, and cook 2 minutes more without stirring so the meat browns.

Pour in the beef stock and red wine, season the sauce with the dried rosemary, 1/4 teaspoon of the salt, and black pepper, and cook 5 to 10 minutes more, stirring occasionally, until the liquid has reduced by half. Slice the pita bread in half and fill each pocket with some of the meat mixture. Garnish with yogurt dressing.

Yield: 6 sandwiches

monterey chicken paninis

I love paninis, and this zesty Southwest version of the sandwich is one of my favorites. While you can toast paninis in a large skillet, the traditional grill marks rendered by an outdoor grill, stovetop grill pan, or electric panini grill create a much more interesting and delectable sandwich.

Ingredients:
1 tablespoon olive oil
4 chicken breast halves, rinsed and dried on paper towels
Coarse salt and freshly ground black pepper, to taste
2 poblano peppers
2 red bell peppers, sliced
1/2 large onion, sliced
4 ounces pepper jack cheese, sliced
1 loaf ciabatta or focaccia bread, sliced into wedges

Preheat a large grill pan over medium heat. When the pan is hot, add the olive oil and swirl to coat the bottom of the pan. Season chicken with salt and pepper and place it in the pan along with the poblano peppers. Cook the chicken 4 minutes, until the bottom side is golden brown, turn the breasts over, and cook 4 minutes more. Turn the meat and cook it 2 minutes more on each side, then transfer it to a platter and cover it to keep it warm.

Continue cooking the poblano peppers, turning them as needed, until they are blistered. Place them in a plastic zipper bag for 5 minutes so that they steam and soften. Then peel and seed them, and cover them to keep them warm. Add bell peppers and onion to the pan and sauté them several minutes until they are crisp-tender.

Slice chicken and poblano peppers, and place them on the bottom half of each wedge of bread. Add red peppers, onions, and cheese, and top with top halves of each wedge of bread. Toast paninis in the grill pan, turning them over once, and flattening them with a cast-iron skillet or burger press as they cook.

Yield: 8 sandwiches

squash blossom, sweet onion, and asadero quesadilla

When you're hungry but have only ten minutes to create something nourishing and tasty, don't stop at the fast-food restaurant. Instead, whip up a quesadilla like the one featured here. It's my own version of a recipe Carol Morales of Morales Farms gave me. Carol's farm is in Granby, Colorado, and I like to visit her booth when she comes to Dillon's farmers market with her fragrant herbs and fresh greens.

Tender squash blossoms are sautéed with a thick slice of sweet onion, and layered between flour tortillas with juicy, ripe tomato and Asadero cheese. The tortilla is heated in the skillet until it's just toasted and the cheese is melted for a yummy meal in ten short minutes. Who says you don't have time to cook?

Ingredients:
1 tablespoon olive oil
1 thick slice sweet onion
4 fresh squash blossoms, rinsed, stems removed
Coarse salt and freshly ground black pepper, to taste
2 (6-inch) flour tortillas
4 to 5 slices Asadero cheese
3 slices ripe tomato

Preheat a skillet over medium heat, add the olive oil, and swirl to coat the bottom of the pan. Add the onion, sauté 3 to 4 minutes until it begins to brown, and add squash blossoms. Cook 2 minutes more, stirring constantly, until the squash blossoms are heated through and tender. Season lightly with salt and pepper.

Place a flour tortilla on a cutting board, add slices of cheese and tomato, and top with onion and squash blossoms. Place the second tortilla on top and place the entire quesadilla in the skillet. Cook 2 minutes, or until the bottom of the tortilla is golden brown. Turn it over and cook 1 minute more.

To serve, transfer the quesadilla to a cutting board, quarter it, and enjoy!

Yield: 1 sandwich

stuffed burgers with roasted peppers, blue cheese, and caramelized onions

There's only one word to describe these burgers: decadent. Each burger is stuffed with roasted red peppers and tangy blue cheese, topped with sweet caramelized onions, creating a medley of flavors and textures in every bite. Look for jars of roasted peppers in the supermarket aisle with the olives.

Ingredients:
2 tablespoons olive oil
3 large sweet onions, peeled and sliced
2 pounds ground chuck or ground sirloin
1 (8-ounce) jar roasted red bell peppers
4 ounces blue cheese
Coarse salt and freshly ground black pepper, to taste
4 Kaiser rolls or hamburger buns

Heat a large skillet over medium heat, add the olive oil, and swirl to coat the bottom of the pan. Add the onions and sauté until they are golden brown, stirring occasionally, about 10 to 15 minutes. Remove the caramelized onions from the heat and cover them to keep them warm.

While the onions sauté, preheat the grill. Form ground chuck into 8 patties, about 1/4-inch thick. Place a large strip of roasted pepper and several slices of blue cheese on 4 of the patties. Cover each with the remaining 4 patties, pressing the edges well with your fingers to seal in the peppers and cheese. Season the stuffed patties with salt and pepper.

When the grill is hot, cook the burgers over medium heat 4 minutes on each side. Turn them over and cook 3 minutes more on each side, or until they are cooked to the desired degree of doneness.

Place burgers on Kaiser rolls and top them with caramelized onions.

Yield: 4 sandwiches

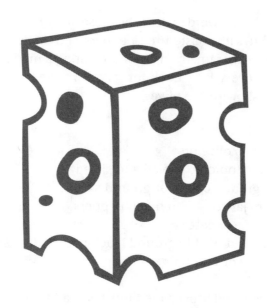

salads, side dishes, and vegetables

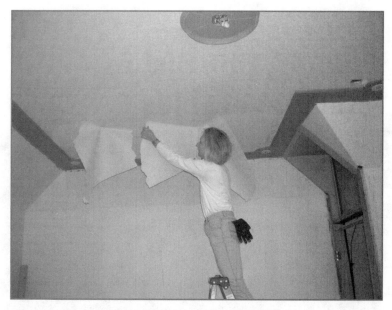

Too Late To Turn Back Now
Removing the artificial "tin ceiling" wallpaper sounded like a good idea until I discovered the mess underneath. Unfortunately, pasting the paper back on was not an option. I should have listened to Randy.

salads

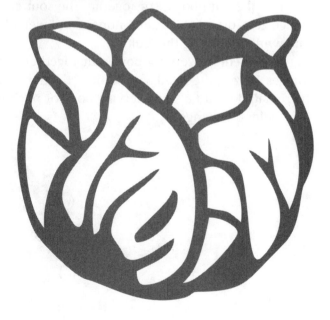

apple and grape salad with honey-orange dressing

This is a scrumptious way to incorporate more fruit in your diet. I've used just-harvested Akane apples—a cross between Jonathan and Red Delicious—in this recipe, but any of your favorites will work well. You'll love the honey-orange dressing on this and other fruit salads.

Ingredients:
1/2 cup nonfat sour cream
1 tablespoon mayonnaise
1 tablespoon orange zest
1 1/2 tablespoons freshly squeezed orange juice
1 tablespoon honey
2 Akane apples, or your favorite eating apple,
  cored and chopped
1 cup green grapes
1 cup red seedless grapes
1 orange, peeled and sliced into bite-size pieces

In a medium bowl, stir together the sour cream, mayonnaise, orange zest, orange juice, and honey until well blended. Cover and chill while preparing the fruit.

In a medium serving bowl, stir together apples, grapes, and oranges. Drizzle the salad with some of the honey dressing and pour the remainder into a small serving bowl or pitcher.

Yield: 6 servings

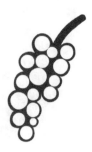

apple and green cabbage slaw

This colorful salad is packed with flavor and nutrition. Cabbage is high in phytochemicals, which, according to the National Cancer Institute, contain cancer-fighting properties. This salad stays fresh in the refrigerator for a couple of days and is ideal for family meals, picnics, and casual summer gatherings.

Ingredients:
1 small head cabbage, shredded or thinly sliced
2 carrots, peeled and grated
2 Red Delicious or other firm red apples, cored and chopped
1/4 cup chopped red onion
1/4 cup white balsamic raspberry vinegar
3 tablespoons canola oil
1 tablespoon sugar
3/4 teaspoon celery seeds
1/2 teaspoon coarse salt
1/4 teaspoon finely ground black pepper
   or peppercorn mélange
1 slice red onion, separated into rings, for garnish (optional)

In a large mixing bowl, stir together the cabbage, carrots, apple, and red onion.

In a small bowl, whisk together the vinegar, canola oil, sugar, celery seeds, coarse salt, and pepper. Pour the vinegar mixture over the cabbage mixture and toss well. Cover and chill until ready to serve.

Just before serving, transfer the salad to a serving bowl and garnish with red onion rings, if desired.

Yield: 8 to 10 servings

beef and black bean taco salads

After years of living in the Lone Star State, I love Tex-Mex food, and if I don't get my Tex-Mex fix at least twice a month, I go into serious withdrawal. When I want a light meal and crave something Tex-Mex, I prepare taco salad. It's spicy, not too filling, and fun to eat. All I need to top it off is a great margarita.

Ingredients:
4 (10-inch) flour tortillas (or taco salad shells)
Nonstick cooking spray
1 1/2 pounds ground chuck or ground sirloin
1 small onion, peeled and chopped
2 cloves garlic, peeled and minced
1 tablespoon taco seasoning
1/4 cup picante sauce
Freshly ground black pepper, to taste
1 small head Romaine lettuce, chopped
1 (15-ounce) can black beans, drained and rinsed
2 ripe avocados, seeded and cubed, or 1 1/2 cups guacamole
2 tomatoes, chopped
1 medium jalapeño pepper, sliced, optional
1/2 cup low-fat or nonfat sour cream

Preheat the oven to 350°F. Spray the tortillas on both sides with nonstick cooking spray and fit them into 7-inch-diameter ovenproof bowls. Place a loosely gathered ball of foil in the center of each tortilla and bake 8 minutes, or until the edges turn light brown. Remove the foil and bake 5 additional minutes, or until the centers are crisp. Transfer the tortillas to a wire rack to cool.

Heat a large skillet over medium heat and add the ground beef and onion. Cook until the meat crumbles and is no longer pink and the onion is translucent. Drain the fat and stir in the garlic, taco seasoning, picante sauce, and pepper. Cook, stirring constantly, 1 minute more.

Divide the chopped lettuce, cooked beef, black beans, avocado, tomatoes, and jalapeño among the four tortilla bowls. Top with a dollop of sour cream. Serve immediately.

Yield: 4 servings

---

fresh spinach and pink grapefruit salad

Tangy, pink grapefruit and sweet, chewy dried cherries team up in this refreshing salad. While you may wish to use fresh grapefruit when they're at the peak of their juiciness, canned grapefruit sections work beautifully and save time. The grapefruit vinaigrette provides a nice counterpoint to both the sweet and sour aspects of this salad.

Ingredients:
1 bunch fresh spinach, washed and dried
1 (15-ounce) can pink grapefruit sections, drained,
   juice reserved
1/3 cup dried cherries
1 teaspoon Dijon mustard
2 tablespoons reserved grapefruit juice
2 teaspoons red wine vinegar
3 tablespoons canola oil
1/4 teaspoon coarse salt
Freshly ground black pepper, to taste
Dash of sugar

Remove the large center stem from the back of the spinach leaves and divide the spinach among four individual salad plates. Place grapefruit sections on top of the spinach and garnish with dried cherries.

In a small bowl, whisk together the Dijon mustard, grapefruit juice, red wine vinegar, canola oil, salt, pepper, and sugar until the dressing thickens. Drizzle the dressing over the salads and serve.

Yield: 4 servings

heirloom tomatoes and spinach
with kalamata olives and shaved parmesan

Juicy heirloom tomatoes, with their irregular shapes and varied colors of red, orange, yellow, and purple, play a starring role in this salad. I like to mix the colors, sizes, and shapes of tomatoes as I arrange this salad, for a rustic, fresh-from-the-country look. Layered on top of fresh spinach leaves, the tomatoes are complemented by kalamata olives, Parmesan shavings, and a drizzle of olive oil and balsamic vinegar.

Ingredients:
1 bunch fresh spinach, washed and dried
2 to 3 heirloom tomatoes of varied colors, sliced
1/2 to 3/4 cup Kalamata olives, pitted
Coarse salt and freshly ground black pepper, to taste
2 to 4 tablespoons olive oil
4 to 8 teaspoons balsamic vinegar
Parmesan cheese

Remove the large center stem from the back of the spinach leaves and divide the spinach among 2 to 4 individual salad plates. Arrange the tomato slices on top of the spinach, garnish with kalamata olives, and season with salt and pepper.

Drizzle each salad with 1 tablespoon of the olive oil and 2 teaspoons of the balsamic vinegar. Hold a wedge of Parmesan cheese in one hand, and with a vegetable peeler, create 1-inch long thin shavings of cheese. Garnish each salad with several shavings.

Yield: 2 to 4 salads

mandarin sesame chicken salad

Crunchy romaine lettuce and chow mein noodles, tender strips of white meat chicken, and sweet mandarin oranges are featured in this Asian-inspired main dish salad. Precooked chicken breasts make this salad particularly quick and easy, or you can sauté or braise chicken breasts just before assembling the salad. A fresh fruit salad and fortune cookies complete the meal.

Ingredients:
2 cloves garlic, peeled and diced
1/3 cup canola oil
2 tablespoons soy sauce
Freshly ground black pepper, to taste
2 tablespoons sesame seeds, toasted and cooled
3 boneless cooked chicken breast halves, sliced into strips
1 bunch romaine lettuce, rinsed, drained, and torn
1 (15-ounce) can mandarin oranges, drained, juice reserved
1 cup chow mein noodles
1/4 cup peanuts

In a small bowl, whisk together garlic, canola oil, soy sauce, and freshly ground pepper until it is well blended. Set aside.

Preheat oven to 250°F. Spread the sesame seeds on a baking sheet and toast them 2 to 3 minutes in the preheated oven; set aside to cool.

Place the lettuce in a large serving bowl, top with the chicken strips and mandarin oranges, and sprinkle with the toasted sesame seeds, chow mein noodles, and peanuts. Drizzle with the Oriental dressing and toss lightly to mix.

Yield: 4 to 6 servings

pear and goat cheese salad with raspberry-champagne vinaigrette

This gorgeous salad of fresh pears, sliced goat cheese, and delicate rose-colored vinaigrette over a bed of greens only looks labor intensive. It's so easy that you'll want to serve it often and so pretty that you'll pull it out for company, too. The combination of sweet, juicy pears and tangy goat cheese is a feast for your taste buds. For added convenience or when fresh pears aren't available, substitute canned sliced pears for fresh. There's no need to sauté them.

Ingredients:
2 pears, peeled, cored, and halved
1 tablespoon unsalted butter
1/4 cup plus 3 fresh raspberries, divided
2 tablespoons raspberry vinegar
1/4 cup champagne
1/2 cup olive oil
Pinch of sugar
Coarse salt and freshly ground black pepper, to taste
1 small bunch salad spring mix, rinsed and spun dry
2 ounces goat cheese

Slice pears to within 1/2 inch of the stem area and gently fan out the slices. In a large skillet over medium-low heat, melt the butter. Add the pears and cook them 4 to 5 minutes until they are tender. Gently transfer them to a platter and set them aside.

In a small bowl, crush 3 of the raspberries with a fork until they are smooth. Whisk together crushed raspberries, raspberry vinegar, champagne, and olive oil until they are well blended. Season with sugar, salt, and freshly ground pepper and stir to mix.

To assemble the salads, place one pear fan on each salad plate. Place a small serving of spring mix to the side of the pears, top with a slice of goat cheese, and drizzle the greens with vinaigrette. Garnish each plate with fresh raspberries.

Yield: 4 servings

salad greens with raspberries, roasted beets, and blackberry balsamic dressing

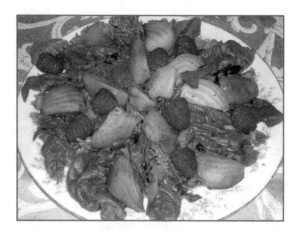

Visually, this is a beautiful salad. I fashion a bed of mixed salad greens and artistically garnish it with plump red raspberries and fresh beet wedges. I like to use yellow and white beets for this recipe, as the red ones stain the other ingredients—and my hands. The beets are best when served cold, so I roast them the day before, cover, and chill them overnight. When sliced into wedges, their natural pattern creates added visual interest.

Blackberry balsamic vinegar is an integral part of this salad, so I've listed purchasing information for it in the "Resource" section. Its complex flavor complements the tart raspberries and roasted beets, and creates a taste experience worthy of slow savoring.

Ingredients:
2 to 3 small to medium yellow or white beets
2 tablespoons olive oil
1 bunch mixed salad greens
1 cup fresh raspberries
1 teaspoon Dijon mustard
1 tablespoon blackberry balsamic vinegar
Coarse salt and freshly ground black pepper, to taste
1/4 cup canola oil

85

One day before you plan to serve the salad, preheat the oven to 350°F. Trim leaves from the beets, leaving a 3-inch stem. Do not trim the roots. Pour olive oil into a large roasting pan, add the beets, and shake the pan to coat the beets in oil. Roast the beets 40 to 45 minutes, or until they are tender. Cool, transfer to a plastic zipper bag, and chill overnight.

Arrange salad greens on a large platter. Using a sharp knife, cut the stems and roots from the beets and peel off the skin. Slice the beets in half, and then into bite-size wedges. Arrange the wedges on top of the salad greens and garnish with raspberries.

Place mustard in a small bowl and pour in balsamic vinegar. Season with coarse salt and pepper, and whisk in canola oil until it is just blended. Drizzle the dressing over the salad and serve immediately.

Yield: 4 to 6 servings

summer fruit salad with sweet and tart dressing

If you love poppy seed dressing, you'll love my quick and easy version, which captures the flavor of this much-loved classic without all the fuss. Let's face it: the shelf life of poppy seeds isn't particularly lengthy, poppy seed dressing requires a lot of oil, and who wants to clean a blender at the end of the day? So, here's a simple, blush-pink dressing that's flavorful, sweet, but slightly tart, to highlight the flavors of summer-fresh cantaloupe, blueberries, and strawberries. I mound the fruit on individual servings of organic baby Romaine or spring mix, to provide added texture and nutrition. During the winter, try this dressing on grapefruit and other citrus salads. You'll love it!

Ingredients:
1 bunch organic baby Romaine or spring mix,
    rinsed and spun dry
2 cups cantaloupe, cubed
1 cup strawberries, sliced or quartered
1 cup blueberries or blackberries
1 tablespoon sugar
1 tablespoon red wine vinegar
A dash of salt
1/8 teaspoon onion powder
1/4 cup canola oil

Divide the salad greens among 4 salad plates and top with the cantaloupe, strawberries, and blueberries or blackberries.

In a small mixing bowl, whisk together the sugar, vinegar, salt, and onion powder until well mixed. Slowly add oil, whisking constantly, until the dressing is thick and creamy. Drizzle it over the salads and serve immediately.

Yield: 4 servings

tomatoes and artichokes with basil

With the availability of juicy vine tomatoes and fresh basil in most markets year-round, you can enjoy this salad anytime. Its attractive appearance and quick preparation make this tasty, nutritious side dish one of my favorites. Add a few grindings of peppercorns mélange for a distinctive flavor.

Ingredients:
4 medium vine-ripened tomatoes, rinsed
1 (14-ounce) can quartered artichoke hearts, drained
2 stems fresh basil leaves
2 to 3 tablespoons olive oil
1 1/2 tablespoons red wine or balsamic vinegar
Coarse salt and freshly ground peppercorn mélange, to taste

Slice tomatoes in half and slice each half into 3 wedges. Place tomato wedges in a medium mixing bowl, add artichokes, and set aside.

Remove the leaves from 1 stem of basil, coarsely chop them, and add them to the tomatoes. Discard the stem. Remove the basil leaves from the second stem and sprinkle the whole leaves over the tomatoes.

Drizzle olive oil and vinegar over the tomato mixture and season with salt and peppercorn mélange. Toss gently and serve immediately, or cover and chill until ready to serve.

Yield: 4 to 6 servings

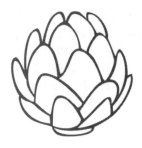

tropical spinach salad with raspberry-poppy seed dressing

This versatile, tropical salad is quick and easy but so pretty, you'll want to keep the recipe on hand for entertaining. I love the vibrant colors and blend of sweet and tangy flavors. For ease of preparation, use canned pineapple and prewashed, packaged spinach and salad greens. Add variety by using your favorite fruits or what's freshest in the market. The raspberry dressing takes just minutes to whirl up in the blender and will stay fresh in the refrigerator for several weeks.

Ingredients:
1 bunch fresh spinach, washed, dried, and stemmed
1 bunch salad greens
2 mangos, peeled and sliced
2 papaya, peeled and sliced
1 cup canned or fresh pineapple
1/2 cup jicama, cut into julienne
1/2 cup sugar
1 teaspoon dry mustard
1/2 teaspoon coarse salt
1/4 cup red raspberry vinegar
1 1/4 tablespoons sweet onion, diced
3/4 cup canola oil
1 teaspoon poppy seeds

On a large platter or individual salad plates, arrange the fresh spinach, salad greens, mango, papaya, pineapple, and jicama.

In a blender, combine the sugar, dry mustard, salt, raspberry vinegar, and onion. Cover and mix on low speed until just blended. With the blender on low speed, add the canola oil slowly in a steady stream until the dressing is thick and emulsified. Add the poppy seeds and pulse several times to mix.

Spoon the dressing over the salad. Extra dressing may be poured into a jar, covered, and stored in the refrigerator for several weeks.

Yield: 4 to 6 servings

wedge salad with red wine–parmesan dressing

Iceberg lettuce wedge salads are popular in Texas steakhouses, and no wonder. They're crisp, cool, and ready in minutes. All that's needed is a dynamite dressing, and my recipe for creamy Parmesan dressing is so scrumptious, you'll want to try it on other salads, too.

Ingredients:
1 tablespoon sugar
1/2 teaspoon dry mustard
1/4 teaspoon coarse salt
1/4 teaspoon freshly ground black pepper
1/8 teaspoon onion powder
1/4 cup red wine vinegar
1 tablespoon mayonnaise
2/3 cup olive oil
1/4 cup Parmesan, finely grated
1 head Iceberg lettuce

In a medium mixing bowl, stir together the sugar, dry mustard, salt, pepper, and onion powder. Add the red wine vinegar and mayonnaise and stir well. Whisk in olive oil and Parmesan until the dressing thickens.

Slice lettuce into 4 or 6 wedges and divide them among individual salad plates. Drizzle with dressing and serve immediately.

Yield: 4 to 6 servings

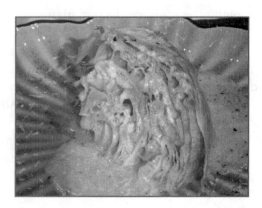

side dishes

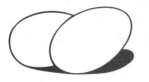

deviled eggs

Add fun to an everyday meal by transforming it into a picnic. Even in the middle of winter, a checked tablecloth on the dinner table, burgers or chicken, purchased potato salad, and a platter of luscious deviled eggs turns an ordinary indoor meal into a holiday gathering. Multicolored peppercorns and capers add a tasty twist to this much-loved classic recipe.

Ingredients:
6 hard-cooked eggs, peeled and sliced in half lengthwise
3 tablespoons mayonnaise
1 to 2 tablespoons nonfat sour cream
1 teaspoon Dijon mustard
1 tablespoon capers, rinsed and drained
Coarse salt and freshly ground black pepper
   or peppercorn mélange
1/4 teaspoon paprika
Fresh parsley for garnish

Remove the egg yolks with a spoon, transfer them to a small mixing bowl, and mash them with a fork. Add mayonnaise, sour cream, and Dijon mustard; stir until well blended. Gently stir in capers, salt, and pepper until just mixed.

Fill egg whites with yolk mixture and sprinkle with paprika. Garnish each egg with a small leaf of parsley and chill until ready to serve.

Yield: 12 deviled eggs

brown rice with apples, dates, and golden raisins

I confess I've never been a real fan of brown rice. I know it's good for me, but it always seemed lacking of flavor. Well, I fixed that! The flavors in this recipe surprised even me, and now I'm a huge fan of brown rice. Apples, dates, and golden raisins team up with fragrant shallots and crunchy walnuts to completely transform brown rice into what may become a favorite side dish in your house. It is in mine.

Ingredients:
1 1/2 cups chicken broth
1 cup water
1 cup brown rice
1/4 teaspoon coarse salt
1 tablespoon olive oil
1 apple, cored and chopped
1 large shallot, peeled and minced
1 stalk celery, diced
1/3 cup golden raisins
1/3 cup chopped walnuts
2 tablespoons chopped dates

In a medium saucepan, stir together the chicken broth, water, rice, and salt, and bring the mixture to a boil over high heat. Cover, reduce heat to medium-low, and cook 45 to 55 minutes, or until the rice is tender and all the liquid has evaporated; set aside and keep warm.

Preheat a large skillet over medium heat, add olive oil, and swirl to coat the bottom of the pan. Add apple, shallots, celery, raisins, walnuts, and dates, and sauté 5 minutes until all are tender.

Add the rice to the sautéed mixture and stir to combine well. Spoon the rice into a large serving bowl and serve.

Yield: 6 servings

brown rice medley with pancetta

A medley of savory flavors and textures takes brown rice from ordinary to extraordinary in this easy-to-prepare side dish. Put the rice on to boil when you first arrive home, then sauté the pancetta, pine nuts, and aromatic vegetables during the final minutes of meal preparation. The pairing of crunchy pine nuts, salty pancetta and olives, and chewy grains of rice makes this dish outstanding.

Ingredients:
1 1/2 cups chicken broth
1 cup water
1 cup brown rice
1/4 teaspoon coarse salt
1 tablespoon olive oil
1 ounce thinly sliced pancetta, chopped
1/2 cup chopped red onion
1/2 cup chopped red bell pepper
1/4 cup green Manzanilla olives with pimientos, halved
2 tablespoons pine nuts
2 tablespoons chopped fresh parsley

In a medium saucepan, stir together the chicken broth, water, rice, and salt, and bring the mixture to a boil over high heat. Cover, reduce the heat to medium-low, and cook 45 to 55 minutes, or until the rice is tender and all the liquid has evaporated; set aside and keep warm.

Preheat a large skillet over medium heat, add the olive oil, and swirl to coat the bottom of the pan. Add the pancetta, red onion, and bell pepper, and sauté 3 to 4 minutes until the vegetables are soft. Add the olives, pine nuts, and parsley, and cook 1 minute more.

Add the rice to the sautéed mixture and stir to combine well. Spoon the mixture into a large serving bowl and serve.

Yield: 6 servings

couscous with green onions and toasted almonds

Couscous, a Mediterranean tradition, is one of my favorite side dishes because it cooks in a matter of minutes. This tiny semolina grain pairs beautifully with a vast array of fruits, nuts, vegetables, and seasonings to create an unlimited selection of accompaniments to any meal. Here, I've paired couscous with scallions and toasted almonds. The dish is ready to serve in 15 minutes.

Ingredients:
1 tablespoon olive oil
5 green onions, green and white parts, sliced
3 tablespoons slivered almonds
1 cup chicken stock or broth
1/4 teaspoon coarse salt
3/4 cup plain couscous

Preheat a medium saucepan over medium heat, add the olive oil, and swirl to coat the bottom of the pan. Add the green onions and almonds, and cook until the almonds are lightly toasted, stirring frequently.

Add the chicken stock and salt, cover, and bring to a boil. When the liquid boils, stir in the couscous, cover, and remove the pan from the heat. Set it aside 5 to 10 minutes until all the liquid is absorbed. Just before serving, fluff the couscous with a fork.

Yield: 4 servings

new potato salad with sugar snap peas and creamy dill dressing

When it's hot outside, this refreshing chilled salad is perfect for lunch or dinner. Add cooked chicken or shrimp to make a complete meal. When I'm pressed for time, I like to cook the potatoes a day ahead so it's a simple matter of steaming the sugar snap peas and whisking up the creamy dressing the next day.

Ingredients:
2 pounds small red potatoes
1/2 pound sugar snap peas
1/4 cup red onion, diced
1/2 cup mayonnaise
5 tablespoons half-and-half
2 teaspoons red wine vinegar
1 teaspoon Dijon mustard
1/4 teaspoon coarse salt
1/8 teaspoon white pepper
1/8 teaspoon paprika
2 tablespoons fresh dill, minced

In a large pot, cook the potatoes over medium heat in enough water to cover until they are fork tender. Drain and set aside to cool. In a medium saucepan, bring sugar snap peas to a boil in 1/2 inch of water, reduce the heat to medium-low, and cook the peas 2 minutes or until they are crisp-tender. Immediately transfer them to a large bowl of ice water to stop the cooking process.

Slice the potatoes into quarters and place them in a large bowl. Drain the snap peas and add them to the potatoes with the onion. Set aside.

In a medium mixing bowl, whisk together mayonnaise, half-and-half, vinegar, Dijon mustard, salt, white pepper, paprika, and dill. Pour the dressing over the potatoes and toss gently to mix. Cover and chill 1 hour or overnight.

To serve, transfer the potato salad to a large platter or serving bowl and garnish with additional dill, if desired.

Yield: 8 servings

roasted red potatoes with rosemary

Tender cubed potatoes are oven-roasted with fresh garlic, fragrant rosemary, and a drizzle of olive oil in this easy side dish. When you're in a hurry, precook the potatoes one day, chill them overnight, and finish them in the oven the next. Serve leftover potatoes for breakfast with eggs.

Ingredients:
10 medium-size red potatoes
3 tablespoons olive oil, divided
3 large cloves garlic, peeled and chopped
Coarse salt and freshly ground black pepper, to taste
1 sprig fresh rosemary, coarsely chopped,
    or 2 teaspoons dried rosemary

Preheat oven to 350°F. Place the potatoes in a large pot and cover with water. Bring the water to a boil, reduce heat to medium-low, cover, and cook until the centers of the potatoes are almost cooked through, about 15 minutes. Drain, slice the potatoes into 1-inch cubes, and set aside.

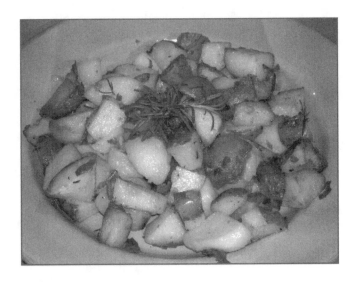

Pour 2 tablespoons of the olive oil into a roasting pan and place it in the oven for 2 minutes, until the oil is hot. Remove the pan from the oven and tilt the pan to distribute the oil evenly. Add the garlic and potatoes, sprinkle them with salt, pepper, and rosemary, and toss.

Drizzle the remaining olive oil over the potatoes and return them to the oven. Roast 20 to 25 minutes, stirring occasionally, until the potatoes are tender when pierced with a sharp knife and the edges are golden brown. Remove the potatoes from the oven, transfer them to a serving bowl, and serve.

Yield: 4 to 6 servings

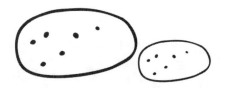

skillet-browned potatoes

If you're a big fan of French fries but are trying to maintain a healthy diet, try these skillet potatoes the next time you're tempted to pull into a fast-food drive-thru lane. Cubed red potatoes are sautéed in a touch of olive oil with lots of garlic and onions until they're golden brown and are finished off with a sprinkle of coarse salt and ground pepper. Dip the finished potatoes into ketchup or enjoy them straight up. With a total preparation time of under 30 minutes, you can enjoy these "fries" anytime.

Ingredients:
4 large (about 1 pound) red potatoes, rinsed
2 tablespoons olive oil
1/4 cup chopped onion
3 cloves garlic, peeled and minced
Coarse salt and freshly ground pepper mélange

Cut the potatoes into 1-inch cubes and place them in a saucepan with enough water to cover them. Bring them to a boil over high heat, reduce the heat to medium-low, and cook them until they are just tender and a sharp knife easily pierces the flesh, about 10 to 12 minutes.

Preheat a large skillet over medium heat, add the olive oil, and swirl to coat the bottom of the pan. Add the potatoes and onion, toss to coat the vegetables with oil, and sauté them about 5 minutes, stirring only after the potatoes start to brown on the bottom. Add the garlic and sauté 5 to 10 minutes more, stirring occasionally, until the potatoes are golden brown. Season them with salt and pepper and serve.

Yield: 4 servings

whipped potatoes

Most adults and kids love whipped potatoes, and thankfully, they are quick and easy to prepare. Their creamy texture and buttery flavor go well with roasts, steaks, chops, and chicken. Topped with a dab of butter or molded into a "bird's nest" and filled with gravy, whipped potatoes are a perfect way to round out a menu.

Ingredients:
2 pounds Russet or Yukon gold potatoes, peeled and cubed
1 teaspoon coarse salt, plus more to taste
Freshly ground black pepper
2 to 3 tablespoons butter
1/4 cup hot milk

Place the potatoes in a large saucepan with enough water to cover them and add 1 teaspoon of the salt. Cover and bring the water to a boil, reduce the heat to low, and boil gently until a sharp knife easily pierces the potatoes, about 10 minutes.

Drain well, reserving the potato water for gravy, if desired. Place the saucepan back on the hot burner for 1 minute, uncovered, to steam off any remaining water. Place the saucepan on a heat-proof surface, season the potatoes with salt and pepper, and whip them with an electric mixer until they are smooth.

Melt the butter in hot milk and pour some of the milk mixture into the potatoes. Beat the mixture on high speed, adding the remaining milk a little at a time, until the potatoes are light and fluffy. Check the seasonings, transfer the potatoes to a serving bowl, and serve.

Yield: 4 servings

white beans, arugula, and dill with tarragon dressing

As a salad or side dish, this medley of creamy white beans, peppery arugula, and delicate fresh dill in a tarragon dressing is a refreshing change of pace. Serve it cold during the summer or at room temperature any time of the year. For an easy main dish salad, top it with slices of grilled chicken.

Ingredients:
2 (15-ounce) cans Great Northern beans, rinsed and drained
3 sprigs fresh dill, chopped
1 small bunch fresh arugula, stemmed and chopped
1/2 cup onion, diced
2 tablespoons tarragon vinegar
2 to 3 drops white wine Worcestershire sauce
1 large clove garlic, peeled
1/2 teaspoon Dijon mustard
Coarse salt and freshly ground black pepper, to taste
1/4 cup olive oil

In a large mixing bowl, gently stir together the beans, dill, arugula, and onion. Set aside.

In the bowl of a mini food processor, combine the tarragon vinegar, Worcestershire sauce, garlic, Dijon mustard, salt, and pepper. Process until the mixture is smooth. Add the olive oil and process until the dressing is creamy. Taste and adjust the seasoning, if necessary. Pour the dressing over the beans. Toss well, transfer the salad to a serving bowl, and serve. If desired, cover and chill 2 hours until cold.

Yield: 6 servings

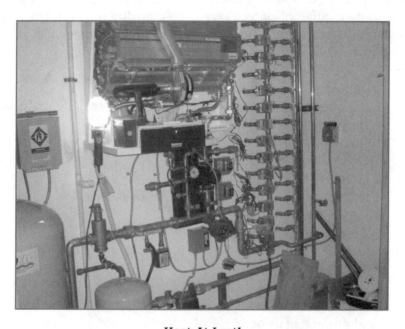

Heat At Last!

After four months of working in a freezing house, with outdoor temperatures sometimes dipping to 17 degrees, our new state-of-the-art boiler makes all the difference.

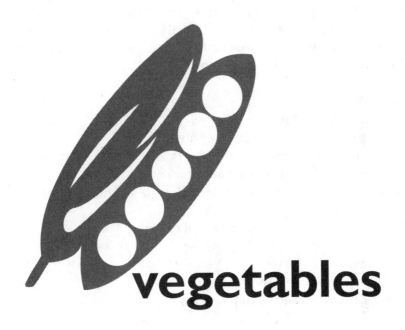

vegetables

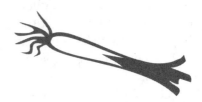

bok choy, sugar snap peas, and fig balsamic stir-fry

I've discovered a line of flavored balsamic vinegars that enable me with no fuss to provide additional layers of flavor to main dishes, salads, and desserts. In this recipe, fig balsamic vinegar adds richness to an otherwise classic vegetable stir-fry. Look for information on flavored balsamic vinegars in "Resources."

Ingredients:
1 tablespoon canola oil
1/4 pound sugar snap peas, trimmed
3 green onions, green and white parts, sliced in 1/2-inch lengths
3 large cloves garlic, peeled and minced
1 1/4 pounds bok choy, green and white parts, sliced at an angle
1 teaspoon cornstarch
1/4 cup vegetable or chicken stock or broth
2 tablespoons fig balsamic vinegar
1 tablespoon soy sauce
1/4 teaspoon coarse salt
Freshly ground black pepper, to taste

Preheat a wok or large skillet over medium heat, add the oil, and swirl to coat the bottom of the pan. Add snap peas, green onion, and garlic, and sauté 1 minute, stirring constantly. Add bok choy and cook 2 to 3 minutes more, stirring constantly. Vegetables should be crisp-tender.

Place cornstarch in a small bowl and whisk in vegetable stock to form a slurry. Pour the mixture into the wok and add fig balsamic vinegar and soy sauce; stir to combine well. Season the vegetables with salt and pepper, and serve.

Yield: 4 to 6 servings

brussels sprouts with tarragon and parmesan cheese

I've zipped up the flavor and aroma of these tiny cool-weather cabbages with a generous sprinkling of fresh tarragon and shaved Parmesan. Tarragon's distinctive anise-like flavor can easily overwhelm more delicate foods but is pleasantly assertive in this particular side dish.

Ingredients:
1 pound fresh brussels sprouts
1 tablespoon olive oil
1 tablespoon butter
2 tablespoons chopped hazelnuts or sliced almonds
2 large cloves garlic, peeled and minced
3 tablespoons chopped fresh tarragon
Coarse salt and freshly ground black pepper
1/4 cup Parmesan, shaved or coarsely grated

Rinse and trim the tough ends from the brussels sprouts. Place the sprouts in a saucepan with enough water to cover them. Cover and bring to a boil over high heat, reduce the heat to low, and simmer 10 to 12 minutes until the vegetables are tender and a sharp knife easily pierces them; drain.

Preheat a large skillet over medium heat, add olive oil and butter, and swirl to coat the bottom of the pan. Add the brussels sprouts and hazelnuts, and sauté, stirring frequently, until the brussels sprouts begin to brown slightly and the hazelnuts are toasted. Add the garlic and tarragon, season well with salt and pepper, and sauté one minute more.

Transfer the brussels sprouts to a serving bowl and garnish with shaved Parmesan cheese.

Yield: 4 servings

butternut squash with apple-date filling

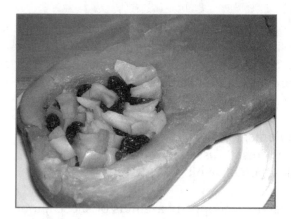

This autumn and winter vegetable dish is simple enough for everyday cooking, but it's so impressive, you may want to serve it when guests join you for dinner. There's no advance sautéing or oven baking. Instead, the squash is steamed on the stove in a large covered skillet, and when tender, the brown sugar–apple filling is mounded into the squash cavity and steamed until it's done. Butternut squash never looked so pretty.

Ingredients:
1 (3-pound) butternut squash, cut in half lengthwise
1 apple, cored and chopped
2 tablespoons dates
1 tablespoon raisins
2 tablespoons brown sugar
2 tablespoons butter

Cut the butternut squash in half lengthwise and scoop out seeds. Fill a large cast-iron skillet with 1/2 inch water and place the squash in the water, cut side down. Cover and bring the water to a boil, reduce the heat to medium-low, and steam the squash 20 to 25 minutes until it is knife tender. Take care not to overcook the squash, as this will cause it to lose its shape.

When the squash is done, turn it over with a metal spatula and fill each cavity with half of the apple, dates, raisins, brown sugar, and butter, layering each ingredient one atop the other. Cover the pan and steam the squash 10 minutes more, or until the apples are soft when pierced with a knife.

Transfer the squash to a serving platter and serve immediately.

Yield: 6 to 8 servings

---

corn on the cob with cilantro butter

I've taken corn on the cob and zipped it up with a zesty melted butter sauce. A mixture of chili powder, crushed red pepper flakes, a bit of salt, and fresh cilantro combine to create robust flavor. Just pour the sauce into a bowl and serve with a small pastry brush. Let everyone brush as much butter sauce on their corn as they like. No more "chasing" after that little pat of butter as it slides off the knife.

Ingredients:
4 ears fresh corn, steamed or grilled
1/2 cup unsalted butter
1 tablespoon fresh cilantro, finely chopped
1/2 teaspoon coarse salt
1/4 teaspoon chili powder
1/8 teaspoon crushed red pepper flakes

Melt the butter in a small saucepan over low heat. When it has melted, add the cilantro, salt, chili powder, and red pepper flakes. Cook 5 minutes, stirring occasionally, to allow the flavors to meld.

To serve, pour the butter sauce into a small bowl and brush it onto the corn. Alternatively, divide the sauce into 4 individual corn-shaped plates and roll the corn in the sauce.

Yield: 4 servings

green beans with apple-smoked bacon

These sweet-and-sour string beans remind me of a dish my mother often made when I was growing up, but I've updated the recipe with serving suggestions and the flavor with apple-smoked bacon. The beans are tasty served hot or cold, so during the cooler months, serve them as a warm side vegetable and, during the summer, their crunchy texture adds variety to cold salad plates.

Ingredients:
3/4 pound green beans, rinsed and trimmed
3 strips apple-smoked bacon, cut into 1-inch pieces
1/4 cup water
1/4 cup cider vinegar
3 tablespoons sugar

Steam the green beans in a steam basket in a saucepan filled with 1/2 inch water until they are crisp-tender, about 5 minutes (or 10 to 12 minutes at high altitude). Transfer them to a serving bowl and set aside.

Cook the bacon in a large skillet until it is crisp, transfer it to paper towels, let it cool, crumble it, and set it aside as a garnish.

Add the water, cider vinegar, and sugar to the hot skillet. Cook 3 minutes over medium heat, stirring to loosen brown bits from the bottom of the pan. Remove the pan from the heat, strain the dressing through a fine sieve, and pour it over the beans. Toss to mix well and garnish with crumbled bacon.

Yield: 4 servings

grilled tomatoes and zucchini

Grilling brings out the flavor of many vegetables, so when I fire up the grill for meats or seafood, I always add vegetables to the mix during those last few minutes of cooking. Two of my favorite veggies to grill are tomatoes and zucchini. They take only minutes to cook and their flavors and colors complement each other. Why not give it a try the next time you cook out?

Ingredients:
3 large tomatoes
3 zucchini
1/4 cup olive oil
Coarse salt and freshly ground black pepper, to taste
Parmesan cheese, grated, optional

Place a vegetable grill basket on the grill and preheat it. While it is heating, slice the tomatoes into thick slices and slice the squash lengthwise. Brush the tomatoes and squash with olive oil and sprinkle them with salt and pepper.

Place the tomatoes and squash on the grill, cook 2 to 3 minutes until they start to brown, and turn them over. Cook 1 minute more and transfer them to a serving platter. If desired, sprinkle with Parmesan cheese, and serve.

Yield: 4 servings

sautéed asparagus with toasted almonds

A zesty citrus dressing and crunchy toasted almonds dress up steamed asparagus for everyday dining. A Microplane zester saves time when garnishing the asparagus with fresh lemon zest. You can, alternatively, use a potato peeler to create long, thin strips of lemon peel as a garnish.

Ingredients:
1 pound fresh asparagus, rinsed
1 tablespoon olive oil
3 tablespoons sliced almonds
1 teaspoon Dijon mustard
1 tablespoon freshly squeezed lemon juice
1/4 cup extra-virgin olive oil
Coarse salt and freshly ground pepper, to taste
1 teaspoon lemon zest, for garnish

Remove the woody end of each asparagus spear by holding the spear in both hands and breaking it. It will snap at the point where the asparagus is tender. Fill a large skillet with water to a depth of 1/4 inch. Place trimmed asparagus in the skillet, cover, and cook over medium-high heat just until the asparagus is crisp-tender, about 2 minutes, depending on the spears' thickness. Drain, set the vegetables aside, and keep warm.

Dry the skillet with a paper towel and place it over medium-low heat. Add the olive oil and swirl it to coat the bottom of the pan. Add the sliced almonds and sauté them 1 to 2 minutes until they are toasted, stirring often. Transfer them to a small plate to cool and set aside.

In a small bowl, whisk together mustard, lemon juice, and extra-virgin olive oil until the mixture is thick and emulsified. Season with salt and pepper.

Return the asparagus to the skillet and place the pan over medium-low heat. Add 1 tablespoon of the lemon vinaigrette and toss well to coat each spear. When the asparagus is hot, transfer it to a serving platter and garnish with lemon vinaigrette, toasted almonds, and lemon zest.

Yield: 4 servings

white asparagus with honey-tarragon vinaigrette

I always purchase white asparagus when I see it in the market because it reminds me of a memorable meal my husband, his parents, our young sons, and I enjoyed just after visiting the chateau at Fountainbleu, while we were living in France. Our younger son, Bob, was about eighteen months old then, and since the restaurant had no high chair for him, he sat in his stroller while we dined, completely enthralled by the restaurant's cat, who took up temporary residence under our table.

The first course was chilled white asparagus with a light and velvety vinaigrette. It tasted divine and our enjoyment of it will forever be connected to watching our little son peeking under the tablecloth throughout the meal.

Ingredients:
1 pound white asparagus, rinsed and woody ends removed
1 teaspoon honey mustard
1 tablespoon tarragon vinegar
3 tablespoons extra-virgin olive oil
1/8 teaspoon coarse salt
Freshly ground pepper mélange
1 sprig fresh tarragon, leaves removed and coarsely chopped

Place the asparagus in a large skillet, fill the pan with water to a depth of 1/4 inch, cover, and bring to a boil over high heat. Immediately reduce the heat to medium-low and simmer the asparagus 3 minutes, or until they are crisp-tender. Drain, set them aside, and keep warm, or, if preferred, transfer them to a plate, cover, and chill them 1 hour or overnight.

In a small bowl, combine honey mustard, tarragon vinegar, olive oil, salt, pepper mélange, and fresh tarragon. Whisk until the dressing is very thick and emulsified. To serve, arrange the spears side by side on individual salad plates and spoon some of the vinaigrette across the middle of the spears.

Yield: 4 servings

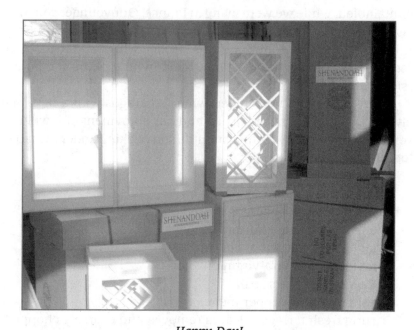

Happy Day!
*After months of designing, changes, and anticipation, our
gorgeous cabinetry for the old kitchen and gold vault arrived on
a very cold winter day. Here, it's stacked and ready for installation.*

desserts

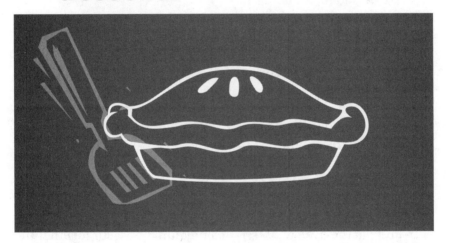

quick apple cobbler with lemon-rosemary drop biscuits

This recipe uses canned apple pie filling, so it's easy to substitute cherry, blueberry, or peach to suit your mood or menu. Covering the cobbler are lemon drop biscuits—so light and tender, with a subtle flavor of fresh rosemary. Delicious!

Ingredients:
2 (21-ounce) cans apple pie filling
4 tablespoons plus 2 teaspoons sugar, divided
1/2 teaspoon cinnamon
1/8 teaspoon allspice
1/8 teaspoon freshly grated nutmeg
1 1/2 cups flour
1 teaspoon baking powder
1/2 teaspoon baking soda
1/4 teaspoon salt
1/4 cup cold unsalted butter, cut into 8 pieces
2 teaspoons lemon zest
1 teaspoon finely chopped fresh rosemary
2/3 cup buttermilk
Vanilla ice cream, optional

Preheat the oven to 350°F. In a medium bowl, stir together the pie filling, 2 tablespoons of the sugar, cinnamon, allspice, and nutmeg until well blended. Pour the mixture into a 9-inch casserole or baking pan and set aside.

In a large bowl, stir together the flour, 2 tablespoons of the sugar, baking powder, baking soda, and salt until well blended. Cut cold butter into the flour mixture with a pastry blender or 2 knives until the butter is pea-size. Quickly stir in the lemon zest, rosemary, and buttermilk until the biscuit dough is light and fluffy.

Drop large dollops of dough onto the apple mixture and sprinkle the biscuits with the remaining sugar. Bake the cobbler 30 to 35 minutes, or until the filling is hot and bubbly and the biscuits are puffy and golden brown. Remove the pan from the oven and set it aside to cool.

Serve the cobbler warm or at room temperature with a scoop of vanilla ice cream, if desired.

Yield: 6 to 8 servings

---

cranberry-apple country tart

The beauty of a rustic country tart is its free-form shape, which many find easier to create than a traditional pie. Just drape the almond pastry onto a baking sheet or into a pie plate, spoon in the filling, and gather up the pastry around the filling. What could be easier? If you're short on time, use premade pie pastry, which you can find in most supermarkets. Either way, this pretty fruit tart is sure to please your family and friends. Look for information about sparkling sugar in "Resources."

Ingredients:
1/3 cup thinly sliced almonds
1 1/2 cups plus 1 tablespoon flour, divided
1/2 cup plus 1 1/2 tablespoons sugar, divided
1/2 teaspoon salt
1/2 cup cold unsalted butter, cut into 8 pieces
3 tablespoons ice water
1/4 teaspoon almond extract
3 to 4 baking apples, peeled, cored, and sliced
1 cup fresh cranberries
1 teaspoon cinnamon
1/2 teaspoon freshly grated nutmeg
2 teaspoons fresh lemon juice
1 egg
1 tablespoon water
1 tablespoon sparkling sugar or 2 teaspoons
  granulated sugar, for garnish

Place the almonds in the bowl of a food processor and process until they are finely ground. Add 1 1/2 cups of the flour, 1 1/2 table-spoons of the sugar, and the salt, and pulse several times until the ingredients are mixed.

Add cold butter and pulse until the butter is pea-size. Add ice water and almond extract, and process until the pastry comes together and forms a ball. Do not overprocess. Remove the pastry, wrap it in plastic wrap, and chill it at least 30 minutes or until it is cold.

While the pastry is chilling, preheat the oven to 400°F. In a large bowl, stir together apples and cranberries. In a small bowl, mix the remaining sugar, the remaining flour, the cinnamon, and the nutmeg. Pour the sugar mixture into the cranberries and apples, add the lemon juice, and toss well to mix.

On a floured pastry cloth, roll the chilled pastry into a 14-inch circle. Fold the pastry in half and transfer it to a baking sheet covered with parchment paper. Unfold the pastry and fold the edges of the paper up to catch any juices that may overflow during baking.

Pour the filling into the center of the pastry, mounding it in the center, and fold the edges of the pastry up around the filling, over-lapping the edges to form a round tart. Take care the pastry doesn't tear around the base of the tart or juices will escape during baking. The center of the tart should remain open.

In a small bowl, whip the egg and water together with a fork. Brush the egg wash over the pastry and sprinkle it with sparkling or granulated sugar. Bake in a preheated oven 30 to 35 minutes, or until the pastry is golden brown and the apples are tender when pierced with a sharp knife.

Yield: 1 tart

brandied apple crisp with trail mix crumble

This is the dessert I make when it's chilly outdoors and I want something that will fill the house with the fragrance of cinnamon. It's also the perfect recipe when I want a quick dessert, and there are only a few apples in the crisper. The crisp looks fabulous when baked in individual ramekins, but you can also prepare it in a 9-inch baking pan. The trail mix crumble topping is crunchy and incredibly flavorful, making this one of my favorite no-fuss recipes.

Ingredients:
4 crisp apples, such as Gala or Granny Smith
6 (6-ounce) ramekins or custard cups
1/4 cup dried cherries
2 tablespoons raisins
1 1/2 tablespoons brandy
2/3 cup granulated sugar
1 tablespoon cornstarch
1 teaspoon cinnamon
1/4 teaspoon ground cloves
1/4 teaspoon freshly grated nutmeg
3/4 cup Post Grape-Nuts Trail Mix Crunch cereal
1/4 cup quick-cooking oats
2 tablespoons brown sugar, packed
3 tablespoons butter, melted

Preheat the oven to 375°F. Peel, core, and slice the apples directly into the ramekins and set them aside.

In a small saucepan over low heat, combine the cherries, raisins, and brandy. Cook the mixture 3 to 4 minutes, stirring occasionally, until the fruit is plump and the brandy is absorbed. Sprinkle the brandied fruit over the apples.

In a small bowl, combine the granulated sugar, cornstarch, cinnamon, cloves, and freshly grated nutmeg. Divide the mixture evenly between the ramekins, spooning the mixture directly over the apples.

In a medium bowl, stir together the trail mix cereal, oats, brown sugar, and melted butter until the mixture is moist, and sprinkle it over the apples. Place the ramekins on a large cookie sheet lined with parchment paper and bake in a preheated oven 30 minutes, or until the juices are bubbly and the apples are tender when pierced with a sharp knife. Serve the dessert warm or at room temperature.

Yield: 6 servings

---

almond toffee brickle bars

When you need to bake something for school or the office, these two-layer cookie bars are quick and easy. Press the almond toffee dough into the bottom of a pan, bake, and sprinkle on the butterscotch crumb topping. After a few more minutes in the oven, they're ready to slice and enjoy. Positively scrumptious!

Ingredients:
1 cup unsalted butter, softened
1 cup granulated sugar, divided
1 1/4 cups light brown sugar, packed, divided
1 egg yolk
1/2 teaspoon vanilla
2 1/4 cups flour, divided
1/4 teaspoon salt
1/2 cup almond toffee bits
1/4 cup graham cracker crumbs
3 tablespoons butter, melted
2/3 cup butterscotch morsels

Preheat the oven to 350°F. In the bowl of an electric mixer, cream the softened butter, 3/4 cup of the granulated sugar, and 1/4 cup of the brown sugar until it is light and fluffy, about 4 minutes. Add the egg yolk and vanilla, and beat until smooth.

In a medium bowl, combine 2 cups of the flour and the salt. Gradually add the flour mixture to the creamed mixture, beating until it forms a soft dough. Stir in the toffee bits. Press the dough into the bottom of a 9x13-inch pan and bake 12 minutes.

While the bottom layer is baking, stir together remaining brown sugar, the remaining granulated sugar, the remaining flour, the graham cracker crumbs, and the melted butter in a medium bowl until the ingredients are moistened. Stir in the butterscotch morsels.

When the bottom layer is baked, remove the pan from the oven, sprinkle the dough evenly with the butterscotch crumb mixture, and return the pan to the oven. Bake 20 minutes more.

Remove the pan from the oven and cool 15 minutes. Slice into bars, remove them from the pan, and cool completely on a wire rack. Store the cookies in an airtight container.

Yield: 16 large bar cookies

acorn squash pie

You can have all the flavor of autumn squash pie without the work by substituting premade piecrust for my homemade pastry. But purists will find this pastry is light and flaky. Just remember, the keys to flaky pastry are using ice-cold ingredients and avoiding over-working the dough. This acorn squash pie is similar to pumpkin pie, just a little lighter and more delicate.

Ingredients:
1 1/4 cups flour
1/4 cup sifted cake flour
1/2 cup plus 1 tablespoon sugar, divided
1 1/2 teaspoons salt, divided
5 tablespoons cold unsalted butter
2 tablespoons shortening
3 to 4 tablespoons ice water
1 very large acorn squash, halved, seeded,
    and steamed until tender
1/2 cup brown sugar, packed
1 teaspoon cinnamon
1/2 teaspoon freshly grated nutmeg
1/2 teaspoon ground ginger
1/4 teaspoon allspice
3 eggs
1 1/2 cups half-and-half

Place the flours, 1 tablespoon of the sugar, and 1/2 teaspoon of the salt in the bowl of a food processor and pulse several times to mix. Slice the butter into 5 pieces and add it to the flour mixture along with the shortening; pulse until the butter is pea-size.

Add 3 tablespoons of the ice water and pulse at low speed until the pastry forms crumbs; add more ice water by the teaspoon if the mixture appears dry. Process on low speed until the pastry comes together and forms a ball. Remove the pastry, wrap it in plastic wrap, and chill it at least 30 minutes or until it is cold.

Roll the pastry out on a floured pastry cloth, trim the edges with a knife, fold it in half, and transfer it to a 10-inch pie plate. Unfold the pastry, fit it into the pie plate, and trim and crimp the edges; set aside. Preheat the oven to 425°F. Scoop the cooked squash from the peel, transfer it to the bowl of a food processor, and process until it is smooth. Transfer the squash to the bowl of an electric mixer and add the remaining granulated sugar, the brown sugar, the remaining salt, cinnamon, nutmeg, ginger, and allspice. Beat on medium speed until the ingredients are just combined.

Add eggs and beat well. Gently whisk in half-and-half until the filling is smooth. Strain the filling through a sieve into the prepared piecrust and bake it 15 minutes. Reduce the oven heat to 350°F and bake the pie an additional 40 to 45 minutes, or until the filling is set and a sharp knife comes out clean when it is inserted into the middle of the filling.

Remove the pie from the oven and set it on a rack to cool. Cover and chill any leftovers.

Yield: 1 10-inch pie

coconut-raisin chewies

Even when I'm extremely busy, I sometimes crave the aroma of homemade cookies in the air, so I'll drop everything and bake a batch of cookies. These cookies are absolutely the best—moist, chewy, and full of oatmeal, raisins, and coconut. Once you try them, I bet you'll stay up late now and then and bake a batch, too.

Ingredients:
Nonstick cooking spray
2 cups flour
1/2 teaspoon baking powder
1/2 teaspoon baking soda
1/2 teaspoon salt
3/4 cup unsalted butter, softened
1/4 cup shortening
1/2 cup granulated sugar
1/2 cup brown sugar, packed
2 eggs
1 teaspoon vanilla
3/4 cup sweetened flaked coconut
3/4 cup quick-cooking rolled oats
1 cup raisins
Additional granulated sugar, for garnish

Preheat the oven to 350°F. Lightly grease cookie sheets with cooking spray. In a medium bowl, stir together the flour, baking powder, baking soda, and salt; set aside.

In the bowl of an electric mixer, cream the butter, shortening, and sugars until light. Add the eggs, vanilla, and coconut and beat until thoroughly mixed.

Using a large spoon, gradually stir the flour mixture into the creamed mixture until well blended. Stir in oatmeal and raisins. Drop generous teaspoons of cookie dough onto the prepared cookie sheets, leaving 2 inches between each one.

Bake 10 to 12 minutes until the cookies are puffed and golden brown. Remove them from the oven, sprinkle with granulated sugar, and transfer them to wire racks to cool.

Yield: 3 1/2 dozen 3-inch cookies

caramel brownies

Just because time is short doesn't mean there's no time for dessert. These decadent, chocolaty brownies have a caramel filling right through the middle. It's like an extra treat in every bite. So get out your spatula and a mixing bowl, and turn on your oven. This dessert snack is worth every minute.

Ingredients:
6 ounces unsweetened chocolate
1 cup unsalted butter
3/4 cup granulated sugar
1/2 cup brown sugar, packed
2 teaspoons vanilla
6 large eggs
1 cup flour
3/4 teaspoon baking powder
1 (14-ounce) bag caramels, unwrapped
3 tablespoons heavy cream

Preheat the oven to 350°F. Place the chocolate and butter in a microwave-safe bowl and microwave 2 minutes on high power, stopping once to stir the ingredients. Remove the bowl from the microwave and stir until the chocolate is melted and smooth.

Stir the granulated sugar, brown sugar, and vanilla into the chocolate mixture. Add the eggs and beat well. Add the flour and baking powder and blend thoroughly. Spoon half of the batter into a 9x13-inch greased pan and bake 12 minutes.

While the brownies are baking, place caramels in a medium saucepan, add cream, and cook over medium-low heat, stirring occasionally, until the caramels have melted and the mixture is smooth. Remove the pan from the heat, set it aside, and keep it warm.

Remove the brownies from the oven, spread warm caramel over them with a rubber spatula, top with remaining brownie batter, and return the pan to the oven. Bake 15 minutes more, or until a cake tester inserted into the center comes out clean. Cool and slice the brownies into squares.

Yield: 1 9x13-inch pan brownies.

grilled pineapple and nectarines

During the summer, when nectarines are ripe and juicy, I love cooking them on the grill with tart, sweet pineapple rings or slices. This simple dessert needs only a sprinkle of brown sugar during the final minute of cooking to become a summer treat you'll look forward to each year.

Ingredients:
3 large nectarines, rinsed
12 pineapple rings or slices, fresh or canned
1/4 cup canola oil
1/2 cup brown or demerara sugar, packed

Preheat the grill. While it is heating, slice nectarines in half, twist to separate the halves, and remove pits. Transfer pineapple and nectarines to a large platter and brush them lightly with oil.

Place the pineapple and nectarines, cut side down, on the grill and cook 3 to 4 minutes, or until the bottoms are golden brown. Turn them over, sprinkle them with brown sugar, and cook 1 to 2 minutes more, or until the brown sugar has caramelized and the fruit is knife tender.

Transfer the cooked fruit to a large platter or shallow bowl and serve hot. If desired, serve fruit with ice cream.

Yield: 3 to 6 servings

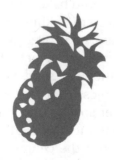

purple gooseberry tarts with cinnamon-sugar puff pastry

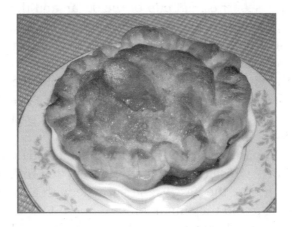

One early September day, as I was shopping at the weekly farmers market in Dillon, Colorado, I spied fresh purple gooseberries in a booth of locally grown salad greens, herbs, and vegetables. Their flavor reminded me of grapes—the perfect starting point for individual deep-dish tarts. I topped each tart with puff pastry, which, when baked, created puffy cinnamon-sugar clouds.

When time is short, but you want an impressive dessert, these purple gooseberry tarts are definitely the answer. Try this basic recipe with sliced purple plums or blackberries when gooseberries aren't in season.

Ingredients:
1 pint purple gooseberries, rinsed (about 2 cups)
2/3 cup plus 1 tablespoon sugar, divided
2 teaspoons cornstarch
1/2 teaspoon vanilla
1 tablespoon unsalted butter
1 sheet frozen puff pastry, thawed
1 egg
1 tablespoon water
1/8 teaspoon cinnamon

Preheat the oven to 375°F. In a medium bowl, gently stir together the gooseberries, 2/3 cup of the sugar, and the cornstarch. Add the vanilla and stir gently until the filling is just mixed. Pour the berry mixture into 6-ounce ramekins or custard cups, dot with butter, and set aside.

Slice the puff pastry into thirds along the fold line, rewrap one section in plastic wrap, and return it to the freezer. Slice the remaining 2 sections in half and roll each out on a floured pastry cloth into a 5 1/2 by 5 1/2-inch square.

Drape the pastry over the ramekins and fold and flute the edges. In a small bowl, whisk the egg and water together to form a pastry wash, brush it over the pastry, and sprinkle with a mixture of the remaining sugar and the cinnamon.

Place the ramekins on a cookie sheet covered with parchment paper, and bake 25 to 30 minutes until the fruit is bubbly and the pastry is puffed and golden brown. Serve warm or at room temperature.

Yield: 4 tarts

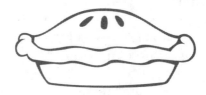

raspberry sorbet trifle

This pretty-in-pink layered dessert can be ready at the drop of a hat, thanks to prepared pound cake. Fresh raspberries are layered with sorbet, blueberry syrup, and cubes of cake to create a quick version of the English trifle. Individual parfait glasses or wine goblets make it easy to prepare only the number of desserts needed, and if you have trouble getting the kids to eat enough fruit, supplement the raspberries with sliced bananas and fresh blueberries or blackberries. Then try to convince them this dessert is good for them.

Ingredients:
2 teaspoons blueberry or blackberry syrup
2 small scoops raspberry sorbet
1/3 cup fresh raspberries
1 slice prepared pound cake, cubed
Whipped cream or whipped topping, optional

Pour 1 teaspoon of the blueberry syrup in the bottom of a 6-ounce parfait glass and top it with a small scoop of sorbet, half of the raspberries, and cubes of cake. Add another scoop of sorbet and the remaining raspberries. Drizzle the trifle with the remaining blueberry syrup and garnish with a swirl of whipped cream, if desired.
Yield: 1 dessert

red plum compote

When plums are ripe and juicy, this compote makes a fabulous low-fat dessert, whether served warm or cold. If you can't resist, it's pretty wonderful over a scoop of ice cream, too. I leave the skins on when I cook the plums because the skins are nutritious and lend a soft pink color to the compote.

Ingredients:
7 large red plums, about 2 pounds, sliced
1/2 cup water
1/2 cup sugar
1 tablespoon red currant jelly

In a medium saucepan, combine the plums, water, and sugar. Bring the mixture to a boil over medium-high heat, reduce the heat to medium-low, and cook, uncovered, 12 to 15 minutes, stirring frequently. The plums should be soft but keep their shape. Stir in the red currant jelly until it melts.

Remove the pan from the heat and set it aside to cool. Serve the plums warm or transfer them to a serving bowl, cover, and chill. Plums may be served alone, with a scoop of ice cream, or with a slice of pound cake or cheesecake.

Yield: 6 to 8 servings

sautéed pears with vanilla–brown sugar sauce

In this recipe, canned or fresh pears are transformed into an elegant dessert in 15 minutes. Pear halves are sautéed in a touch of butter, brown sugar, and pear nectar until they are tender. The addition of a vanilla bean to the sauce adds a noteworthy layer of flavor to this otherwise simple dessert. Serve the pears alone or with a scoop of vanilla or coffee ice cream.

Ingredients:
2 tablespoons unsalted butter
1/2 cup light or dark brown sugar, packed
1 (29-ounce) can Bartlett pear halves or
    6 fresh pears, peeled, cored, and halved
1/4 cup pear nectar
1 vanilla bean or 1/2 teaspoon vanilla extract
1/4 teaspoon freshly grated nutmeg
1/2 cup pecan halves, optional
Vanilla or coffee ice cream, optional

Preheat a large skillet over medium heat and add the butter and brown sugar. Cook the mixture 2 to 3 minutes, or until the brown sugar has melted and is bubbly, stirring constantly.

Reduce the heat to medium-low, arrange the pears, cut side down, in the brown sugar syrup, and cook 2 minutes until they begin to soften. Turn the pears over, add the pear nectar, vanilla bean, nutmeg, and pecans to the pan, and cook 3 to 4 minutes more.

To serve, spoon two halves and some of the sauce into individual shallow bowls and, if desired, top with a scoop of ice cream.

Yield: 5 to 6 servings

spice cupcakes

Everyone loves cupcakes. Cupcakes are uncomplicated, the perfect serving size, and fun to eat. I developed my recipe for spice cupcakes one afternoon when I felt the first cool breezes of an early Colorado autumn and I was craving something sweet. Iced with cream cheese frosting and garnished with a dash of shaved dark chocolate, these cupcakes are the ideal dessert or snack.

Baked goods prepared at a high altitude can taste bland without a boost in flavoring, so you'll notice I've added vanilla to the list of ingredients—you won't need this vanilla if you're at sea level. I've also added a bit more milk for bakers at high altitude so your cupcakes won't be dry.

Ingredients:
1 cup unsalted butter, softened
1 1/4 cups granulated sugar
1/2 cup brown sugar, packed
3 eggs
1 teaspoon vanilla extract (use only if baking at high altitude)
2 1/2 cups flour
1 1/2 teaspoons baking powder
1 teaspoon salt
3/4 teaspoon cinnamon
1/2 teaspoon freshly grated nutmeg
1/4 teaspoon ginger
1/4 teaspoon ground cloves
1 cup milk (add an extra 2 tablespoons milk
    if baking at high altitude)

Preheat the oven to 350°F. In the bowl of an electric mixer, cream the butter and sugars until the mixture is light and fluffy, about 5 minutes. Add the eggs, one at a time, beating well after each addition. If baking at high altitude, stir in the vanilla.

In a medium bowl, stir together the flour, baking powder, salt, cinnamon, nutmeg, ginger, and cloves. Gradually add the flour mixture to the creamed mixture, alternately with the milk, beating well between each addition.

Line two 12-cup muffin tins with paper liners. Spoon the batter into the tins, filling each cup three-quarters full. Bake 18 to 20 minutes until the top of each cupcake is golden and a cake tester inserted into the center of a cupcake comes out clean.

Remove the tins from the oven, and remove the cupcakes from the pans while they're still hot so they don't become soggy. Cool on a wire rack while making the Cream Cheese Frosting.

Cream Cheese Frosting:
1/2 cup unsalted butter, softened
1 (3-ounce) package cream cheese, softened
4 cups confectioners' sugar, sifted
A dash of salt
4 to 7 tablespoons milk
1 teaspoon vanilla
1 bar dark chocolate, for garnish

In the bowl of an electric mixer, cream the butter, cream cheese, confectioners' sugar, and salt, adding milk as needed until frosting reaches a creamy consistency. Stir in the vanilla.

Frost each cupcake with some of the frosting and garnish immediately with shaved chocolate so the chocolate sticks to the frosting. To create chocolate shavings, hold the chocolate bar in one hand over a large plate and shave it with a vegetable peeler. Chocolate shavings are delicate, so use a spoon to scoop up shavings to prevent crushing them with your fingers.

Yield: about 24 cupcakes

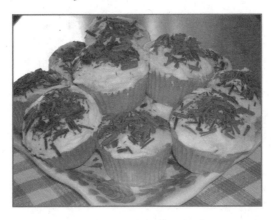

strawberry angel parfait

This gorgeous strawberry parfait is worthy of a magazine cover. Fresh strawberries are layered in a parfait glass or wine goblet with low-fat strawberry yogurt, cubes of angel food cake from the bakery department, and raspberry or strawberry syrup. The result is a picture-perfect dessert that goes past your lips but not to your hips. You'll find raspberry or strawberry syrup in the supermarket near the maple syrup or where ice cream toppings are displayed.

Ingredients:
2 teaspoons raspberry or strawberry syrup
1/2 cup sliced strawberries
4 tablespoons low-fat strawberry yogurt
1 slice angel food cake, cubed
1 small whole strawberry, for garnish
Mint leaf, for garnish

Pour 1 teaspoon of the raspberry or strawberry syrup into the bottom of a 6-ounce parfait glass. Top with half of the sliced strawberries, 2 tablespoons of the strawberry yogurt, and the cubes of angel food cake. Top with the remaining sliced strawberries, yogurt, and strawberry syrup. Add a whole strawberry and mint leaf for garnish.

Yield: 1 dessert

strawberries romanoff crepes

Enjoy this easy but extravagant dessert whenever strawberries are ripe and juicy. Use my oh-so-flavorful crepe recipe, or for a dessert in minutes, purchase packaged crepes, found in the produce section of most supermarkets.

Ingredients:
1 quart ripe strawberries, washed and drained
2 tablespoons freshly squeezed orange juice
2 tablespoons Grand Marnier or Cointreau
1/2 cup heavy cream
1 teaspoon confectioners' sugar
2 eggs
1 cup milk
1 cup flour
2 tablespoons sugar
1 tablespoon butter, melted
1 teaspoon vanilla

At least 1 hour before serving, slice the strawberries and place them in a medium bowl. Stir in the orange juice and Grand Marnier, cover the berries with plastic wrap, and chill, stirring occasionally. Whip the heavy cream with the confectioners' sugar until soft peaks form, cover, and chill.

While filling is chilling, lightly grease and preheat a crepe pan or 7-inch nonstick skillet over medium heat. In a medium bowl, whisk together the eggs and milk until they are well blended. Gradually whisk in the flour until the batter is the consistency of heavy cream. Stir in the sugar, melted butter, and vanilla.

When the crepe pan is hot, pour 1/4 cup of the batter into the pan and swirl the pan so the batter coats the bottom in a thin layer. Place the pan back on the heat and cook 30 seconds, or until the edges of the crepe dry slightly and the bottom is light brown. Using a fork to lift the crepe, flip it over and cook it 10 seconds. Then transfer the crepe to a large plate and cover it with a towel. Cook and stack the remaining crepes, keeping them covered with a towel so they don't dry out. Crepes may be wrapped in plastic wrap and chilled up to 2 days.

To assemble, place a crepe, brown side down, on a dessert plate. Spoon marinated berries down the crepe's center and fold one side over the filling. Fold the other side over and top with a swirl of whipped cream.

Yield: 10 7-inch crepes.

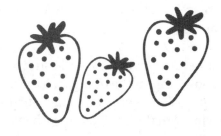

sweet cherry sponge cakes with ricotta cream

Packaged ladyfingers make this dessert quick and easy. Fresh cherries and a brandy marinade make it fabulous. This pretty-as-a-picture dessert looks elegant but is deceptively easy to create for special family celebrations or last-minute dinner guests. Delicate sponge cakes are garnished with marinated fresh cherries and a dollop of sweetened heavy cream and ricotta cheese. Ladyfingers freeze well for several weeks, so keep some on hand for spur-of-the-moment desserts.

Ingredients:
1/2 pound fresh sweet cherries, pitted and halved
3 ounces cherry-flavored or other brandy
2 tablespoons freshly squeezed orange juice
1/2 teaspoon sugar
1 cup heavy cream
2 tablespoons ricotta cheese
1 teaspoon confectioners' sugar
1 (3-ounce) package ladyfingers
Fresh mint sprigs, for garnish

In a small bowl, stir together cherry halves, cherry brandy, orange juice, and 1/2 teaspoon sugar. Cover and chill at least 30 minutes, stirring occasionally.

In the bowl of an electric mixer, whip heavy cream until soft peaks form. Add ricotta cheese and confectioners' sugar, and continue beating until the mixture is well blended.

Place ladyfingers on individual dessert plates and top with marinated cherries and a dollop of ricotta cream. Garnish each dessert with a sprig of mint.

Yield: 6 servings

sour cream–cinnamon muffins

The center of these light, tender muffins, perfect for breakfast or as a special accompaniment to dinner, reveals a layer of fragrant cinnamon sugar. For variety, add shredded apple or fresh blueberries or raspberries to the batter or as a tasty surprise in the middle, then sprinkle the top of each muffin with cinnamon sugar just before baking. Absolutely scrumptious!

Ingredients:
2 cups flour
1 teaspoon baking powder
1 teaspoon salt
1/2 cup unsalted butter, softened
1 1/2 cups granulated sugar, divided
2 eggs
1/2 cup low-fat sour cream
2 teaspoons vanilla
1/2 cup milk
1 teaspoon cinnamon
1/4 teaspoon freshly grated nutmeg

Preheat the oven to 400°F. In a medium bowl, stir together the flour, baking powder, and salt, until thoroughly mixed.

In the bowl of an electric mixer, cream the butter and 1 cup of the sugar until light. Add the eggs and sour cream, beating well after each addition. Stir in vanilla.

Stir flour mixture into creamed mixture, alternating with the milk. In a small bowl, stir together the remaining sugar, cinnamon, and nutmeg; set aside.

Line muffin tins with paper liners or spray with nonstick cooking spray and fill them one-third full. Sprinkle them liberally with some of the cinnamon sugar and top with additional batter until the muffin tins are three-quarters full. Sprinkle the top of the batter with additional cinnamon sugar.

Bake the muffins in a preheated oven 18 to 20 minutes until they are golden brown and a tester inserted into the center comes out clean. Remove the muffins from the oven and transfer them to a wire rack or lined basket. Serve warm.

Yield: 16 muffins

Cook's Note: For high altitude baking, add 2 to 3 tablespoons additional milk and 1 teaspoon additional vanilla to the batter.

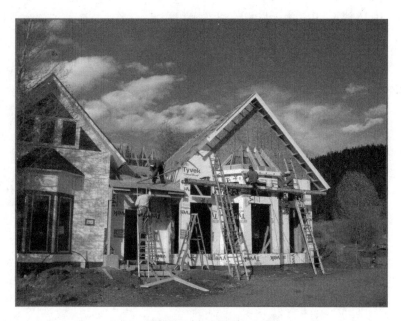

My Dream Kitchen
This will be the kitchen of my dreams, with plenty of counter space,
a huge center island, drawers and cupboards for everything, a fireplace,
and the most breathtaking mountain views I could imagine.
It's a kitchen for cooking, family, friends, and romantic
candlelight dinners with my sweetheart.

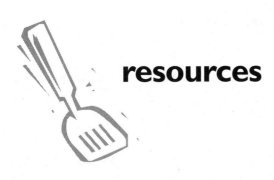

resources

Here is a resource list for some of my favorite ingredients. Please look for the following companies' products in your supermarket or visit their websites.

Cabot Creamery: butter, cheeses, dips, and yogurt
    1 Home Farm Way
    Montpelier, VT 05602
    (888) 792-2268
    www.cabotcheese.com

California Vegetable Specialties: red and white California endive
    15 Poppy House Road
    Rio Vista, CA 94571
    (707) 374-2111
    www.endive.com

Frieda's, Inc.: specialty produce
    Los Alamitos, CA 90720
    (800) 241-1771
    www.friedas.com

India Tree, Gretchen Goehrend & Associates: sparkling sugars, dusting sugars, fondant, herbs, and spices
    Seattle, WA 98119
    (800) 369-4848
    www.indiatree.com

Maille, UNILEVER France: Dijon mustards, oils, and vinegars
    23, rue François Jacob
    92842 Rueil-Malmaison Cedex
    www.maille.com

Melissa's/World Variety Produce: everyday and specialty produce
    PO Box 21127
    Los Angeles, CA 90021
    (800) 588-0151
    www.melissas.com

Mozzarella Company: fresh mozzarella and artisan cheeses
    2944 Elm Street
    Dallas, TX 75226
    (800) 798-2954
    www.mozzco.com

Nielsen-Massey Vanillas: vanilla, vanilla beans, and pure extracts
    1550 Shields Drive
    Waukegan, IL 60085
    (800) 525-7873
    www.nielsenmassey.com

OSO Sweet Onions: the sweetest onions in the world,
available mid January to late March
    www.ososweetonions.com

Pasta Moré Gourmet Foods: flavored balsamic vinegars and oils,
pasta, pesto, and sauces
    7975 E. Harvard Avenue, Unit F
    Denver, CO 80231
    (720) 748-2448
    www.pastamore.com

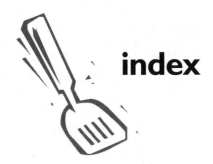

index

about the author

CHRISTY ROST's culinary career began in early 1992, when she became the food editor for a Dallas-area newspaper, and has expanded to include work as an author, television chef, radio personality, guest speaker, entertaining expert, stylist, and spokesperson. She hosts cooking seminars with Macy's, has her own long-running Fort Worth television cooking and lifestyle show, *Just Like Home*, and is a guest chef on countless local and national television shows.

Now she adds two more titles to her resume—historic home owner and restorer. Christy and her husband, Randy, are currently restoring Swan's Nest, the 1898 Breckinridge, Colorado home they purchased as a vacation getaway.

Christy's first cookbook, *The Family Table: Where Great Food, Friends, and Family Gather Together*, introduced readers to one of her passions—gathering families, friends, and neighbors around the table to celebrate daily life and special occasions. Christy is a member of the International Association of Culinary Professionals and a registered nurse. She lives with her husband in Dallas, Texas, and Breckinridge, Colorado. Visit her website: www.christyrost.com.

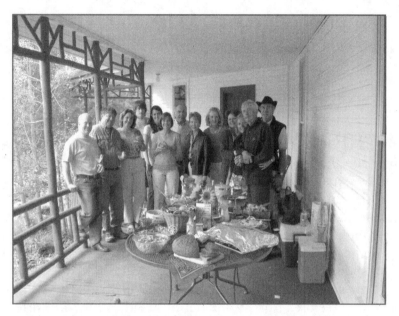

No Kitchen, No Power, But Lots of Friends

*This Labor Day celebration on Swan's Nest's front porch shows
the most important aspect of any gathering is just being together.
If we had waited until the kitchen was remodeled, the electricity
was hooked up, and we had running water, Randy and I would have
missed a delightful afternoon with new friends and neighbors.*